Case Studies in Sleep Neurology

Common and Uncommon Presentat

Case Studies in Sleep Neurology

Common and Uncommon Presentations

Edited by

Antonio Culebras
Suny Upstate Medical University and Community General Hospital, Syracuse, NY, USA

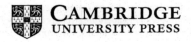

CAMBRIDGE
UNIVERSITY PRESS

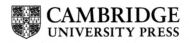

Shaftesbury Road, Cambridge CB2 8EA, United Kingdom

One Liberty Plaza, 20th Floor, New York, NY 10006, USA

477 Williamstown Road, Port Melbourne, VIC 3207, Australia

314–321, 3rd Floor, Plot 3, Splendor Forum, Jasola District Centre, New Delhi – 110025, India

103 Penang Road, #05–06/07, Visioncrest Commercial, Singapore 238467

Cambridge University Press is part of Cambridge University Press & Assessment,
a department of the University of Cambridge.

We share the University's mission to contribute to society through the pursuit of
education, learning and research at the highest international levels of excellence.

www.cambridge.org
Information on this title: www.cambridge.org/9780521146487

First published 2010 (version 2, August 2022)

A catalogue record for this publication is available from the British Library

Library of Congress Cataloging-in-Publication data
    Case studies in sleep neurology : common and uncommon presentations / [edited by] Antonio Culebras.
        p. ; cm.
    Includes bibliographical references and index.
    ISBN 978-0-521-14648-7 (pbk.)
    1. Sleep disorders–Pathophysiology–Case studies.   2. Nervous system–Diseases–Complications–Case
studies.   I. Culebras, A.
    [DNLM: 1. Sleep Disorders–physiopathology–Case Reports.   2. Nervous System Diseases–complications–
Case Reports.   3. Sleep Disorders–etiology–Case Reports.   WM 188]
    RC547.C374 2010
    616.8'49807–dc22

                                                                                                    2010029821

ISBN 978-0-521-14648-7 Paperback

To my fellow torchbearers, who shone the light in multiple directions.

To our faithful readers, who trusted the wisdom of our teachings.

To my family, who patiently accepted the absences.

Antonio Culebras

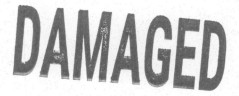

DAMAGED

Contents

Part VIII Neuromuscular disorders and sleep

The following cases described herein have been published previously

Case 24   Adapted from the following publication, with permission from the
publisher: Schenck CH. Uncontrolled intimacy: sexual sleep disorders
[Case report]. *Sleep Review* 2007; 8:24–28.

Foreword

Sleep medicine, for most clinicians, is a new clinical discipline in medicine and one which has appeared almost overnight. To those who thought that all that needed to be known was taught in medical school or in other postgraduate clinical programs, the reality is that very little formal education in sleep medicine has occurred in clinical programs and the clinician is now faced with having to understand the basic science, the underlying physiology and pathophysiology of sleep, and apply that understanding to help diagnose and treat the more than 80 clinical sleep disorders that have currently been described[1]. This book, *Case Studies in Sleep Neurology*, goes a long way in helping the clinician develop the clinical skills to understand, diagnose and treat many of those 80 sleep disorders, but not all, and after reading this book the clinician will be left with an enthusiastic desire to expand his or her knowledge by seeking out and learning about the many additional sleep disorders that could not possibly be covered in this comprehensive volume.

Although all of us sleep on a daily basis and appreciate the importance of full alertness in performing our occupational and social activities, many clinicians, other than those trained in sleep medicine, have little awareness of the importance of sleep and wake issues in the clinical practice of patients with medical, psychiatric and even surgical disorders. Sleep is a function of the brain, yet even in neurology there is still little appreciation of its importance in routine neurological practice. This book helps to highlight some of the neurological aspects of sleep medicine that will aid, not only the sleep specialist, but also the neurologist in managing patients that may have multiple co-morbidities.

Whether one diagnoses one of the most common sleep disorders, such as obstructive sleep apnea syndrome, or one of the more esoteric sleep disorders, such as catathrenia, which is described in this book, the clinician will come to realize that neurological function is an important component of all sleep disorders. Although standard texts on sleep medicine usually provide detailed descriptions of the sleep disorders, in clinical practice patients are more complex, often having multiple medical or psychiatric illnesses, and their clinical course may be complicated by numerous psychoactive medications. The management and course of such patients can only be addressed by books that detail the diagnostic and clinical progress such as described here in *Case Studies in Sleep Neurology*.

Sleep medicine has always been a part of clinical neurology, even before Gélineau described narcolepsy, which some clinicians initially thought could be a psychiatric disorder. Yet to the neurologist, the absence of reflexes during cataplectic attacks confirmed a neurophysiological component to one of the most common disorders of excessive sleepiness. The electroencephalogram, a powerful tool to evaluate neuronal activity, was applied to help understand the underlying physiological basis of sleep and wakefulness, and although partly supplanted by newer diagnostic tests, it is still the basis for determining the cyclical features of the sleep–wake process and is widely utilized in the diagnosis of sleep disorders.

Newer, more advanced electroencephalographic techniques utilizing wider electrode arrays, video, and spectral analysis are helping to clarify both the diagnosis and the central nervous system locations of the effects of sleep and sleep deprivation on the underlying brain. Coupled with analysis of executive function by means of performance tests, studies have shown that the prefrontal cortex (PFC) is a prime area of impairment in sleep loss and excessive sleepiness. Such studies are being applied to many sleep disorders, including the evaluation of both the effects of excessive sleepiness, and the neurotoxic intravascular components of sleep disorders such as obstructive sleep apnea syndrome.

A PubMed search of published articles on neurology and sleep for 2009 revealed nearly 1000 publications suggesting that 2010 will be the decade of advances in the understanding of the brain's role in sleep, wakefulness and sleep loss, as advanced neurological investigative tests involving neurochemistry, neurogenetics and neuroimaging are applied clinically.

The neurochemical control of sleep involves multiple neurotransmitter systems, but most investigations have focused on hypocretin, histamine, dopamine, serotonin and acetylcholine. The recent recognition that the neuropeptide hypocretin is absent in patients with narcolepsy and cataplexy has led to a better understanding of the neurochemical basis of sleep disorders and led to consideration of utilizing neurochemical analysis in establishing sleep diagnoses.[2] In addition, more recently, decreased histaminergic neurotransmission has been shown in narcolepsy and idiopathic hypersomnia, regardless of hypocretin status; the significance of this finding is still unclear.[3] These findings hold promise for new treatments for the sleep disorders that might include hypocretin agonists or histamine H3 antagonists; neurochemical agents that are currently under investigation.

The neurogenetic control of the sleep–wake cycle is an exciting area of future exploration. Numerous genes have been described in animals that influence the sleep–wake cycle and some of these have clinical significance. Some patients with advanced sleep phase syndrome, and more recently some with delayed sleep phase syndrome, have been shown to have an alteration of the period, PER, gene, believed to be a major contributor to the clinical phenotype. Candidate PER3 genes have been discovered that are associated with individual differences in the vulnerability to sleep loss.[4] Future studies that involve candidate genes and neuroimaging may help find biomarkers for neurobehavioral vulnerability to sleep loss and help identify the source of variance in human neurobehavioral responses to sleep deprivation.

Newer, advanced neuroimaging techniques allow for the quantification of a variety of aspects of brain function including brain structure, metabolism, blood flow and receptor binding. These studies have helped understand the brain areas involved in sleep disturbance. Sleep deprivation is associated with global declines in absolute cerebral metabolism as assessed by [^{18}F]FDG positron emission tomography (PET), and regionally these declines are most notable in the PFC and thalamus.[5] These regions have also been shown on functional MRI to be affected by sleep deprivation.[6] Regional cerebral blood flow studies utilizing SPECT scans have shown increased PFC activity that was reversed by chronic administration of modafinil in narcoleptic patients, suggesting that "sleepiness" could result from alterations in the thalamocortical arousal networks that are affected by modafinil therapy.[7]

All of these newer advanced neurological techniques will become more available to the clinician as the research and clinical data grow, and their appropriate role will need to be understood and applied by the sleep medicine clinician.

For most of the abnormal behaviors during sleep such as REM-sleep behavior disorder, sleepwalking, nocturnal frontal lobe epilepsy, rhythmic behavior disorder, and others, video-polysomnography as described in this book is essential to characterize the clinical features of the disorders. Neurochemical analysis of hypocretin has a place in the management of narcolepsy; neurogenetics will play a larger role as our knowledge expands. Many of the clinical cases described in this book, including sleep disorders associated with multiple sclerosis, subdural hematoma, nocturnal frontal lobe epilepsy, and thalamic lesions have utilized newer neuroimaging techniques to aid in the diagnosis.

The clinician can start the process of understanding the role of advanced neurological investigative means and the appropriate clinical management of sleep disorder patients by reading the case histories contained in *Case Studies in Sleep Neurology*.

1. *International Classification of Sleep Disorders*, 2nd edn. Westchester, Illinois: American Academy of Sleep Medicine, 2005.

2. Nishino S, Okuro M, Kotorii N, *et al.* Hypocretin/orexin and narcolepsy: new basic and clinical insights. *Acta Physiol (Oxf)*. 2010; **198**(3): 209–22.

3. Kanbayashi T, Kodama T, Kondo H, *et al.* CSF histamine contents in narcolepsy, idiopathic hypersomnia and obstructive sleep apnea syndrome. *Sleep* 2009;**32**(2):181–7.

4. Groeger JA, Viola AU, Lo JC, *et al.* Early morning executive functioning during sleep deprivation is compromised by a PERIOD3 polymorphism. *Sleep* 2008;**31**:1159–67.

5. Thomas ML, Sing HC, Belenky G, *et al.* Neural basis of alertness and cognitive performance impairments during sleepiness II. Effects of 48 and 72 h of sleep deprivation on waking human regional brain activity. *Thalamus Relat Syst* 2003;**2**:199–229.

6. Chee MW, Choo WC. Functional imaging of working memory after 24 hr of total sleep deprivation. *J Neurosci* 2004;**24**(19):4560–7.

7. Joo EY, Seo DW, Tae WS, *et al.* Effect of modafinil on cerebral blood flow in narcolepsy patients. *Sleep* 2008;**31**(6):868–73.

Michael J. Thorpy MD
Director, Sleep-Wake Disorders Center
Montefiore Medical Center and
Professor of Neurology
Albert Einstein College of Medicine
Bronx, New York

Contributors

Adel K. Afifi MD MS
Professor of Pediatrics, Emeritus, Roy J. & Lucille A. Carver College of
Medicine, University of Iowa, Iowa City, IA, USA

Maha Alattar MD
Neurology Consultant & Sleep Medicine Specialist, Mary Washington Hospital,
Fredericksburg, VA, USA

Ran D. Anbar MD FAAP
Professor of Pediatrics & Medicine Department of Pediatrics, SUNY Upstate
Medical University, Syracuse, NY, USA

Hrayr P. Attarian MD
Associate Professor, Vermont Regional Sleep Medicine Center, Department of
Neurology, University of Vermont College of Medicine, Burlington, VA, USA

Kyoung Bin Im MD
Fellow in Sleep Medicine, The University of Iowa Sleep Disorders Center,
Iowa City, IA, USA

Leslie H. Boyce MD
Assistant Professor, Raleigh Neurology Associates, Raleigh, NC, USA

Elizabeth Budman
Medical Student, SUNY Upstate Medical University, Syracuse, NY, USA

Giovanna Calandra-Buonaura MD
PhD Fellow in Sleep Medicine, Department of Neurological Sciences,
University of Bologna, Bologna, Italy

Teresa Canet PhD
Chief of Neurophysiology Service, Clinical Neurophysiology Department,
Virgen de los Lirios Hospital, Caramatxel, Alcoy, Alicante, Spain

Philip Cherian MD
Senior Neurology Resident, Department of Neurology, SUNY Upstate
University Hospital, Syracuse, NY, USA

Pietro Cortelli MD PhD
Professor of Neurology, Department of Neurological Sciences, University of Bologna, Bologna, Italy

Antonio Culebras MD
Professor of Neurology, Upstate Medical University, and Consultant, The Sleep Center, Community General Hospital, Syracuse, NY, USA

Mark Eric Dyken MD FAHA FAASM
Director, Sleep Disorders Center, Department of Neurology, The University of Iowa Roy J. and Lucille A. Carver College of Medicine, Iowa City, IA, USA

Baruch El-Ad MD FAASM
Sleep Medicine Center, Technion – Israel Institute of Technology, Haifa, Israel

Tik Dion Fung MD
Fellow, Department of Clinical Neurosciences, University of Calgary Foothills Medical Center, Calgary, Alberta, Canada

Michael J. Howell MD
Assistant Professor, Department of Neurology, University of Minnesota Medical Center, Minneapolis, MN, USA

Marcel Hungs MD PhD
Assistant Clinical Professor & Director, Center for Sleep Medicine, Department of Neurology, University of California, Irvine, Orange, CA, USA

Sheldon Kapen MD
Chief, Neurology Section, VA Medical Center and Associate Professor of Neurology, Wayne State University and Veterans Administration Medical Center, Detroit, MI, USA

Lynn V. Kataria MD
Resident in Sleep Medicine, Department of Neurology, University of North Carolina Chapel Hill, NC, USA

Philip King MBBS, MM, FRACP
Discipline of Sleep Medicine, University of Sydney, Sydney, NSW, Australia

Chon Lee MD
Fellow, Department of Neurology, University of North Carolina School of Medicine, Chapel Hill, NC, USA

Deborah C. Lin-Dyken MD
Clinical Associate Professor of Neurology, Development & Behavior,
Center for Disabilities & Development, Department of Pediatrics,
Roy J. & Lucille A. Carver College of Medicine, Iowa City, IA, USA

Mark W. Mahowald MD
Minnesota Regional Sleep Disorders Center and Hennepin County
Medical Center, University of Minnesota Medical School, Minneapolis,
MN, USA

David E. McCarty MD
Assistant Professor, Sleep Medicine Program, Department of Neurology,
Louisiana State University Health Sciences Center, Shreveport, LA, USA

Pasquale Montagna MD
Professor of Neurology, Department of Neurological Sciences, University of
Bologna, Bologna, Italy

Kamal Nasser MD
Wayne State University Medical School, Detroit, MI, USA

Federica Provini MD
Department of Neurological Sciences, University of Bologna,
Bologna, Italy

Cherridan Morrison Rambally MD
Sleep Medicine Fellow, Vermont Regional Sleep Center, Burlington,
VT, USA

Carlos H. Schenck MD
Minnesota Regional Sleep Disorders Center, Hennepin County Medical Center,
University of Minnesota, Minneapolis, MN, USA

Michael H. Silber MD
Professor of Neurology & Co-Director, Sleep Disorders Center, Mayo Clinic,
Rochester, MN, USA

Rosalia C. Silvestri MD
Professor & Director, Sleep Medicine Center, Department of Neurosciences,
University of Messina, Messina, Sicily, Italy

Zafer N. Soultan MD
Assistant Professor of Pediatrics, SUNY Upstate Medical University,
Syracuse, NY, USA

Bradley V. Vaughn MD
Professor of Neurology & Director, Division of Sleep & Epilepsy,
Department of Neurology, University of North Carolina School of Medicine,
Chapel Hill, NC, USA

Roberto Vetrugno MD PhD
Researcher, Sleep Centre, Department of Neurological Sciences,
University of Bologna, Bologna, Italy

Michael J. Zupancic MD
Pacific Sleep Medicine Services, San Diego, CA, USA

Abbreviations

ADHD	attention deficit hyperactivity disorder
ADNFLE	autosomal dominant nocturnal frontal lobe epilepsy
AHI	apnea–hypopnea index
AI	apnea index
BECTS	benign epilepsy with centrotemporal spikes
BID	twice a day
BMI	body mass index
bpm	beats per minute
BRA	benzodiazepine receptor agonist
CAP	cyclic alternating pattern
CBT	cognitive behavioral therapy
CMT	Charcot–Marie–Tooth disease
CPAP	continuous positive airway pressure
CSA	central sleep apnea
CSF	cerebrospinal fluid
CSR	Cheyne–Stokes respiration
CSWS	continuous spike and wave in sleep
CT	computed tomography
ECG	electrocardiogram
EDS	excessive daytime sleepiness
EEG	electroencephalogram
EMG	electromyogram
EOG	electro-oculogram
ET_{CO2}	end-tidal CO_2
FDA	US Food and Drug Administration

GABA	gamma-aminobutyric acid
HIV	human immunodeficiency virus
MMT	methadone maintenance treatment
MRI	magnetic resonance imaging
MSA	multiple system atrophy
MSLT	multiple sleep latency test
NES	nocturnal eating syndrome
NFLE	nocturnal frontal lobe epilepsy
NPD	nocturnal paroxysmal dystonia
NREM	non-rapid eye movement
OSA	obstructive sleep apnea
OSAHS	obstructive sleep apnea–hypopnea syndrome
OSAS	obstructive sleep apnea syndrome
PAMS	periodic arm movements of sleep
PAP	positive airway pressure
PLegMS	periodic leg movements of sleep
PLM	periodic limb movement
PLMA	periodic limb movement while awake
PLMD	periodic limb movement disorder
PLMS	periodic limb movements of sleep
PO	per os (by mouth)
PRN	when necessary
PSG	polysomnography
PSM	propriospinal myoclonus
PtcCO$_2$	transcutaneous CO$_2$
PTSD	post-traumatic stress disorder
QAM	once a day in the morning
QHS	at every bedtime
QPM	once a day in the evening
RBD	REM-sleep behavior disorder

RDI	respiratory disturbance index
REM	rapid eye movement
RLS	restless legs syndrome
RMD	rhythmic movement disorder
SB	sleep-related bruxism
SNRI	selective norepinephrine reuptake inhibitor
SPECT	single-photon-emission computed tomography
SRED	sleep-related eating disorder
SSRI	selective serotonin reuptake inhibitor
TID	three times a day
TST	total sleep time
WASO	wake after sleep onset

Introduction

After a long day roaming the hot plains of Castille, Don Quixote and his faithful squire Sancho Panza decided to call the day off and rest under a lone tree. They shared a meager supper of stale bread, musty cheese from La Mancha and rancid red wine. A few grapes found at the bottom of their satchel topped the repast. Despite the frugality of the meal, Sancho felt the customary post-prandial slumber coming and without further ado fell asleep. It displeased Don Quixote, perpetual insomniac, that Sancho had only but one sleep that lasted him from night till morning. "Look how serene the night is, and how lonely is this place, which invites us to vary one slumber with a little watching. Get up, in Heavens name!" exclaimed Don Quixote. Alarmed, Sancho responded, "I only know that while I sleep I have neither fear, nor hope, nor trouble, nor glory. Good luck to him who invented sleep, the cloak that covers all of man's thoughts, the food that takes away all hunger, the water that quenches all thirst, the fire that warms the cold, the cold that cools the heat, the general coin, in short, with which all things are bought, the balance and weight that levels the shepherd with the king and the fool with the wise man. There is only one bad thing about sleep, as I have heard say, and it is that it looks like death, for between one sleeping and one dead there's mighty little difference."

Chapter LXVIII. Miguel de Cervantes Saavedra. Don Quixote of La Mancha. Translated by Walter Starkie. Published by the New American Library, Inc. New York and Toronto. The New English Library Limited, London, 1957 and 1964.

Sleep is the only free voluptuosity given to humans by Nature. Sleep is as necessary as food or drink. When sleep fails, many other biological functions suffer. Sleep is a function of the brain and the neurology of sleep its corollary. And yet, so numerous are the ramifications and so extensive the reach of sleep and its disorders, that sleep medicine remains a multidisciplinary body at the center of which lies sleep apnea, a pervasive disease that has emerged as a public health problem, as have sleep deprivation, excessive daytime sleepiness and fatigue. In the end, however, the neurology of sleep will prevail as the core discipline underlying sleep functions and dysfunctions, the study of which in the hotbed of the brain will lead to a better understanding of their nature.

With great excitement and enthusiasm, we present this book featuring case studies in sleep neurology. The book presents a series of clinical situations representative of problems that challenge the clinical-solving abilities of practitioners in the neurology of sleep, also known as neurosomnology. The book focuses attention on the major categories of sleep medicine including insomnia, hypersomnias, sleep-breathing disorders, parasomnias and circadian dysrhythmias with emphasis on the neurology of sleep. Both usual and unusual cases are presented with the aim of creating a teaching tool that stimulates the thinking process in sleep neurology along established lines of practice. Each case is introduced with an allusive title, followed by a clinical history, an examination and special studies. This sets the stage for the question asking the diagnosis, treatment or management of the case. The follow-up section states the clinical diagnosis and describes the proper clinical actions to be taken based on the results of tests, with a discussion of the differential diagnosis where appropriate. Each presentation ends with general remarks based on current knowledge and standards of practice. A section entitled "Pearls and gold" summarizes the teaching, take-home points. The bibliography introduces the reader to one or two historical references, where available, followed by a recommended review article, and in all cases to five to ten specific citations. Illustrations have been added where appropriate.

The result is a book containing 40 case histories that provoke and educate clinicians at all stages in their careers. The book is intended to be a didactic tool that dares clinical skills, stimulates memory and provides orientation for additional reading. The target audience is sleep medicine specialists and neurologists. Physicians in training in the discipline of sleep and physicians interested in the knowledge of clinical sleep medicine, with particular curiosity for neurological situations, will find the book singularly readable and useful. The authors are skilled clinicians and seasoned writers with academic titles and vast experience in sleep medicine. As constituents of an international elite in sleep neurology, many are part of that first generation of sleep specialists that has enjoyed the privilege and been granted the unique opportunity of describing new disorders and novel clinical conditions of sleep, contained herein.

Antonio Culebras, MD
Professor of Neurology
SUNY Upstate Medical University
Syracuse, NY, USA

Part I

Sleep-related breathing disorders

Case 1

Opioid-induced central sleep apnea

Kamal Nasser and Sheldon Kapen

Clinical history and examination

A 42-year-old man presented for evaluation of frequent breathing pauses during sleep, which had been witnessed by his wife for 5 years along with intermittent mild snoring. He also reported excessive daytime sleepiness (EDS), but his Epworth Sleepiness Scale score was only 6/24 (see Appendix). He would wake up unrefreshed in the morning with a dry mouth. He also reported having had difficulties initiating and maintaining sleep for 10 years. He was treated with multiple medications with incomplete resolution of his insomnia. He was taking temazepam 7.5 mg to help him to maintain sleep.

He had been going to bed between 1 and 4 am and waking up between 12 and 2 pm. His sleep latency was less than 5 minutes and his average sleep time was 8–9 hours per night, but he reported three to four nocturnal awakenings with no known triggers. He had problems returning to sleep after these awakenings and usually spent his time reading. He would take one unintentional nap per day of around 60–90 minutes' duration and felt refreshed upon awakening. There were no symptoms suggestive of narcolepsy, parasomnias, leg kicking, restless legs syndrome (RLS), nightmares or post-traumatic stress disorder (PTSD). He denied having any motor vehicle accidents or near accidents related to somnolence.

His past medical history revealed depression and resection of a schwannoma abutting on the cervical spinal cord in 1992, leaving him with Brown–Séquard syndrome characterized by motor deficits on the left, leading to use of a cane, and pain and paresthesia on the right side of his body. He also remained with a partially paralyzed diaphragm.

His social history was negative for alcohol or other substance abuse, but he was an ex-smoker and he drank 12 cups of coffee per day. His medications included bupropion 150 mg BID, temazepam 7.5 mg QHS, docusate 50 mg TID PRN, baclofen 30 mg TID, pregabalin 200 mg BID, tramadol 100 mg TID and morphine

Case Studies in Sleep Neurology: Common and Uncommon Presentations, ed. A. Culebras. Published by Cambridge University Press. © Cambridge University Press 2010.

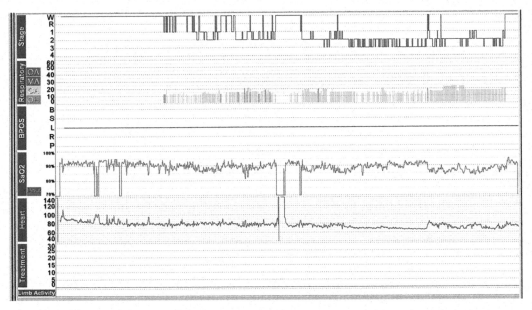

Figure 1.1 Sleep/wake hypnogram of the baseline PSG. Note the severity of central apnea. Central events were prevalent throughout the night (except in the wakefulness stage), with associated O_2 desaturation. OA, obstructive apneas; MA, mixed apneas; CA, central apneas; OH, obstructive hypopneas; BPOS, body position.

sulfate SR 60 mg TID. The patient had been maintained on narcotics for treatment of his chronic pain following the laminectomy, for a period of 8 years. He started with morphine for 3 years, was switched to oxycodone for a few years and then switched back to morphine 5 months prior to his current presentation to the sleep clinic. His family history was negative for obstructive sleep apnea (OSA), narcolepsy, RLS and other sleep disorders. The physical examination revealed a BMI of 18.8 kg/m^2 and an oropharyngeal Mallampati score of 2. He had decreased motor power in the left leg and mild foot drop, and had left arm flaccid paralysis and wrist drop. He was hyperreflexic on the left. He had no other pertinent physical findings.

Special studies and results

In view of his sleep respiratory symptoms, polysomnography (PSG) was performed (Figure 1.1). This revealed a delayed sleep onset (88 min), low sleep efficiency (60.3%) and 340 apneas with an apnea–hypopnea index (AHI) of 89.6 per hour and a central apnea index of 86.8 per hour (Table 1.1). A continuous positive airway pressure (CPAP) titration was scheduled and, after having a discussion with the patient about the potential effects of his medication on

Table 1.1 Summary of the baseline PSG results

Sleep architecture	
Time in bed (min)	390
TST (min)	235
Sleep efficiency (%)	60.3
WASO (min)	58.5
Sleep latency (min)	88
REM sleep latency (min)	N/A
TST supine (min, %)	0 (0)
STAGING	
Stage N1 (min, %)	39 (16.6)
Stage N2 (min, %)	142.5 (60.6)
Stage N3 (min, %)	53.5 (22.8)
Stage REM (min, %)	0 (0)
Respiratory parameters	
Total apneas (no.)	340
Obstructive apneas (no.)	0
Central apneas (no.)	340
Hypopneas (no.)	11
AHI (/h)	89.6
Central apnea index (/h)	86.8
Lowest SaO_2 (%)	81
Waking SaO_2 (%)	91–96

Note: TST, total sleep time; WASO, wake after sleep onset; REM, rapid eye movement; N/A, not applicable; AHI, apnea–hypopnea index.

the results of the obtained sleep study, morphine sulfate was discontinued for 3 months prior to the CPAP titration. A CPAP pressure of 6 cmH$_2$O resulted in complete resolution of the sleep-disordered breathing and improved his sleep morphology (Table 1.2, Figure 1.2).

Question

Why does this patient have central sleep apnea?

General remarks

This case is a good example of opioid-induced central sleep apnea. During the last decade, there has been a marked increase in opioid use following the release of a joint statement from the American Academy of Pain Medicine and the American

Table 1.2 Summary of the CPAP titration results

Sleep architecture	
Time in bed (min)	424.5
TST (min)	302
Sleep efficiency (%)	71.1
WASO (min)	19.5
Sleep latency (min)	103
REM sleep latency (min)	138.5
TST supine (min, %)	0 (0)
STAGING	
Stage N1 (min, %)	16 (5.3)
Stage N2 (min, %)	250 (82.8)
Stage N3 (min, %)	28 (9.3)
Stage REM (min, %)	8 (2.6)
Respiratory parameters	
Total apneas (no.)	0
Obstructive apneas (no.)	0
Central apneas (no.)	0
Hypopneas (no.)	2
AHI (/h)	0.4
Central apnea index (/h)	0
Waking SaO_2 (%)	93–96
Lowest SaO_2 (%)	90% (in NREM)

Note: TST, total sleep time; WASO, wake after sleep onset; REM, rapid eye movement; AHI, apnea–hypopnea index; NREM, non-rapid eye movement.

Pain Society in 1997, which advocated the aggressive use of opioids. This has been accompanied by recognition of the undertreatment of pain and the adoption of pain as another vital sign alongside temperature, heart rate, blood pressure and respiration. Indeed, pain units have now become commonplace in academic centers and community hospitals alike.

Opioid receptors are located in various areas of the brain but particularly in the brainstem where they are found in or around respiratory centers such as the medullary pattern generators and the nucleus of the tractus solitarius. There are three types of opioid receptors: mu, delta and kappa. Most of the opioid medications used for pain control target the mu receptors and these receptors have an inhibitory effect on breathing rate and amplitude.

Although the effects of opioids on waking respiration have long been recognized, awareness of their effects on respiration during sleep is a relatively recent development. Wang *et al.* (2005) studied a group of 50 patients on methadone

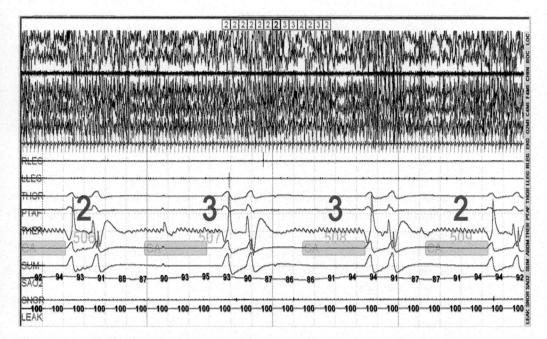

Figure 1.2 A 120-second segment from the patient's PSG study showing a sample of central apneas in stage N2 and N3 sleep associated with significant desaturation. LOC and ROC are left and right electro-oculographic tracings, respectively. Chin EMG is the surface chin electromyographic tracing. F4M1, C4M1 and O2M1 are the right frontal, central and occipital electroencephalographic tracings, respectively. ECG is an electrocardiographic tracing. Airflow tracings by nasal pressure and thermistor are depicted as PTAF and THER, respectively; thorax (THOR) and abdominal (ABDM) movements are also shown along with a pulse oximetry (SAO_2) tracing.

(a mu agonist) maintenance treatment (MMT) and compared them with 20 matched control individuals. Thirty percent of the MMT group and none of the controls had central sleep apnea (CSA), defined as an index of 5 or more events per hour (20% had 10 or more). The obstructive sleep AHI was not different between the two groups. Wang *et al.* (2005) hypothesized that the risk for CSA in the MMT patients was due to an imbalance between central and peripheral chemoreceptors, the former being depressed while the latter were relatively enhanced. This "imbalance" favored the development of CSA because the stimulation of breathing by mild hypoxia will periodically drive CO_2 below the apnea threshold.

Reports of opioid-induced sleep-breathing disorders in populations other than MMT patients have also appeared. Farney *et al.* (2003) described different types of sleep-breathing abnormalities in chronic opioid users including CSA, "ataxic breathing" and sustained hypoxemia. Three patients were symptomatic with fatigue, excessive daytime sleepiness (EDS), sleep disruption and snoring. A larger group of 60 patients who were chronic opioid users was reported retrospectively by Walker *et al.* (2007) and compared with 60 control patients not on opioids. Again, the opioid group had a higher AHI than the controls, almost entirely due to central apneas. The AHI in the opioid subjects was correlated to the morphine equivalent dose and was inversely correlated to the BMI. Of note is that ataxic respiration during sleep was common in the opioid group. Mogri *et al.* (2008) extended the finding of sleep-related CSA to three patients with acute opioid ingestion for relief of non-cancer-related pain. Finally, in a large number of patients attending a pain clinic who had received opioids for 6 months or more, 147 underwent PSG: 24% had CSA, another 8% had CSA together with OSA and 37% had OSA alone. Webster *et al.* (2008) also found a dose–response relationship with CSA, similar to other authors. Thus, these opioid users were similar to MMT patients as far as their sleep-breathing parameters were concerned.

Central sleep apnea is not a common finding in the general population, but nevertheless, several types are recognized besides that induced by opioids. The least common is spontaneous idiopathic CSA, first reported by Guilleminault *et al.* (1973). More common are episodes of CSA that occur at sleep onset in some individuals because of transient fluctuations in the state of consciousness leading to brief arousals accompanied by relative hyperventilation due to CO_2 chemosensitivity. When the subject dozes off, CO_2 levels rise and O_2 levels fall, leading to the arousals that drive the CO_2 levels below the apnea threshold when the subject falls asleep again. The process continues until deeper sleep is attained and no further arousals take place. Finally, there is high-altitude sleep-breathing disturbance characterized by stimulation of overbreathing by hypoxemia and the occurrence of CSA when the apnea threshold is breached. The one factor that these examples of CSA have in common is the importance of the apnea threshold in triggering CSA.

Another form of CSA that has received much attention in recent years is Cheyne–Stokes respiration (CSR). The apnea threshold is also most important in the initiation and persistence of this condition, but it differs from other types of CSA in its phenotypical crescendo–decrescendo manner of breathing following central apneas. Cheyne–Stokes respiration is often associated with congestive heart failure and, when present, there is a higher mortality rate compared with matched heart failure controls with similar ejection fractions. Cheyne–Stokes respiration is also commonly found in patients with supratentorial stroke – in one series, it was present in 50% of patients. However, it is unknown whether it affects the mortality risk in these patients as it does in congestive heart failure.

Several features of our patient are representative of opioid-induced CSA as reported in the literature. One is the patient's BMI ($18.8\,kg/m^2$). The great majority of patients with OSA are overweight or obese; in fact, this is probably the most important risk factor for OSA. On the other hand, several authors have highlighted the opposite trend for opioid-induced CSA (and other forms of CSA); in fact, AHI in CSA seems to be *inversely* proportional to BMI. The reason for this paradoxical association has not been explained in the literature, but one can speculate that there might be an enhancement of peripheral chemosensitivity in thin individuals.

Sleep architecture in opioid users is usually abnormal and, in contrast to patients with OSA, opioid-associated CSA is predominant in NREM sleep whereas obstructive apneas are most often worse during REM sleep. The patient described here had no REM sleep and, consequently, all his respiratory events occurred during NREM sleep. Breathing during NREM sleep (particularly delta sleep, also termed stage N3) is controlled by the metabolic mode of respiration, i.e. blood gases and pH; on the other hand, breathing during REM sleep is largely governed by the "behavioral" mode in which the medullary respiratory centers are under the influence of fibers from higher levels of the brainstem and certain areas of the cerebral cortex. At the same time, the ventilatory responses to CO_2, and to a lesser extent O_2, are depressed in dogs especially, but also in humans, during REM sleep. Other variables, such as those related to the upper airway, are also involved in explaining the dominance of REM sleep in obstructive apneas.

There are no data regarding the outcome of opioid-induced CSA after discontinuation of the offending medication. The patient stopped his morphine 3 months prior to the second PSG study, which was carried out with CPAP, and it can be argued that CPAP was responsible for the improved breathing during sleep.

The management of patients with CSA of whatever cause is uncertain. A number of therapies have been suggested. CPAP was advocated for CSA in the 1980s, only several years following its introduction for the treatment of OSA. The effectiveness of CPAP might be via its role in preventing overbreathing and reduction of CO_2. Another possibility might be stimulation of mechanoreceptors in the upper airway. CPAP has also been investigated as an adjunctive therapy for CSR in congestive heart failure, most notably in the Canadian Positive Airway Pressure study (CANPAP; Bradley *et al.*, 2005).

The trials of pharmacological therapies for CSA have been more variable and less successful. Drugs that have been tried have included theophylline, acetazolamide, serotonergic medications and medroxyprogesterone. The rationale for the use of these drugs differs according to the drug: acetazolamide induces metabolic acidosis, thus stimulating respiratory drive; theophylline inhibits adenosine receptors; medroxyprogesterone stimulates respiration; and clomipramine, a serotonergic uptake inhibitor, is one of a number of serotonergic agonists and antagonists tested for their effects on sleep-related breathing. With the exception of acetazolamide, studies of these medications on CSA have not been encouraging. There is more positive evidence in favor of the use of O_2 in CSA, however. It probably works by eliminating the hyperventilatory response to hypoxia, thus preventing CO_2 from being driven below the apnea threshold. The addition of CO_2 would act in a similar vein, but its administration is less feasible than that of O_2.

Pearls and gold

Non-obstructive forms of sleep-disordered breathing are less common than the obstructive variety. They include upper-airway resistance syndrome, obesity–hypoventilation syndrome, CSR, high-altitude sleep-breathing disorder and CSA, both idiopathic and opioid-induced.

Opioid-induced CSA has attracted attention in recent years because of the surge in opioid administration to patients with pain.

Contrary to OSA subjects, patients with CSA tend to have a low BMI.

SUGGESTED READING

Bradley TD, Logan AG, Kimoff RJ, *et al.* Continuous positive airway pressure for central sleep apnea and heart failure. *N Engl J Med* 2005; **353**: 2025–33.

Farney RJ, Walker JM, Cloward TV, Rhondeau S. Sleep-disordered breathing associated with long-term opioid therapy. *Chest* 2003; **123**: 632–9.

Guilleminault C, Eldridge FL, Dement WC. Insomnia with sleep apnea: a new syndrome. *Science* 1973; **181**: 856–8.

Mogri M, Khan M, Grant B, Mador, J. Central sleep apnea induced by acute ingestion of opioids. *Chest* 2008; **133**: 1484–8.

Walker JM, Farney RJ, Rhondeau SM, *et al.* Chronic opioid use is a risk factor for the development of central sleep apnea and ataxic breathing. *J Clin Sleep Med* 2007; **3**: 455–61.

Wang D, Teichtahl H, Drummer O, *et al.* Central sleep apnea in stable methadone maintenance treatment patients. *Chest* 2005; **128**: 1348–56.

Webster LR, Choi Y, Desaih H, Grant BJ. Sleep-disordered breathing and chronic opioid therapy. *Pain Med* 2008; **9**: 425–32.

Fourteen-year-old with sleep-disordered breathing and excessive daytime sleepiness

Leslie H. Boyce

Clinical history

CF was a 14-year-old young woman who, according to her parents, has had problems sleeping for several years. They reported that at night she would periodically stop breathing and then resume with a loud snorting sound. This would occur multiple times at night and the family felt the need to reposition the child on her side to improve her breathing. She had excessive daytime sleepiness (EDS), and several times a week fell asleep in class. She got into bed at 10–10.30 pm, fell asleep immediately and woke at 7 am. She did not complain of fragmented nocturnal sleep. Occasionally she napped during the afternoon. There were no symptoms consistent with cataplexy, no loss of tone with emotional stimuli and no sleep-onset paralysis or hypnagogic or hypnopompic hallucinations. She reported that her legs occasionally hurt and it helped to move about, but this manifestation was not worse in the evening. There was no history of nocturnal stereotypical movements, sleepwalking or sleeptalking.

Past medical history was notable for preterm birth at 28 weeks' gestation with a birthweight of 4 lbs; birth was via cesarean section secondary to premature rupture of the membrane. She required ventilatory support for less than 24 hours and remained in the hospital for 10 days with some initial feeding difficulties, but was discharged home with no further problems. No other significant medical conditions were present, and her motor and language developments were normal. She had been diagnosed with dyslexia and language-based learning disability, but was able to perform well in school with additional time. There were no symptoms suggestive of attentional deficits or hyperactivity.

The family history was notable for an 11-year-old brother with occasional nocturnal enuresis, and both parents snored but neither had been evaluated for sleep apnea. There was no history of parasomnias, restless legs syndrome (RLS) or neurological disorders. Her parents were divorced and she lived with her mother.

Case Studies in Sleep Neurology: Common and Uncommon Presentations, ed. A. Culebras. Published by Cambridge University Press. © Cambridge University Press 2010.

Examination

Her weight was 46 kg, her BMI was 17.7 kg/m^2 and her vital signs were normal. A general physical examination was likewise normal, with 1+ tonsillar enlargement. A detailed neurological examination was normal.

Special studies

The patient underwent overnight polysomnography (PSG) and an MRI of the head.

Question

What is your differential diagnosis?

Results of studies

Overnight PSG gave the following results (Figure 2.1): sleep latency 4 minutes; sleep efficiency 98%; sleep stage percentages: 5.46% stage N1, 49.28% stage N2, 22.89% stage N3, 22.37% REM sleep.

The patient had a total of 144 sleep-related respiratory events, with an apnea–hypopnea index (AHI) of 22.47 per hour. There were 140 central apneas and four hypopneas, with 126 events occurring in NREM sleep. Minor positional differences were noted, with an AHI of 18 in the lateral decubitus position. The O_2 saturation nadir was 91% and maximal end-tidal CO_2 (ET_{CO2}) was 49 torr.

An MRI of the head (Figure 2.2) showed Chiari 1 malformation with caudal herniation of the cerebellar tonsils through the foramen magnum and resultant crowding at the cranio-cervical junction.

Diagnosis

The diagnosis was Chiari 1 malformation with associated central sleep apnea. The patient also had a syrinx from C3 through the thoracic cord.

Follow-up

The patient underwent suboccipital decompression. She remained in the hospital for 4 days, with some immediate post-operative sleep-related apneas but subsequent significant improvement of sleep. At follow-up, the mother stated that she no longer heard gasping or nocturnal pauses. Daytime sleepiness had disappeared

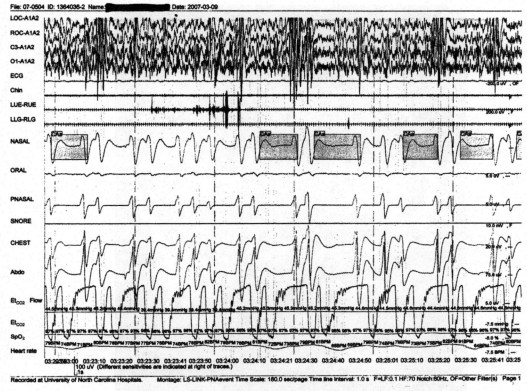

Figure 2.1 Polysomnogram showing frequent central apneas with desaturations. LOC/ROC, left/right outer canthus; LUE/RUE, left/right upper extremity; LLG/RLG, left/right leg; Abdo, abdomen; SpO₂, arterial oxyhemoglobin saturation.

and her schoolwork had improved. A repeat polysomnogram 8 months after surgery revealed a normal study, with only four central apneas throughout the night, giving an apnea index (AI) of 0.48 per hour.

General remarks

Central sleep apnea (CSA) is defined in children under the age of 18 years as a sleep-related respiratory event associated with absent inspiratory effort throughout the entire duration of the event and either (1) lasting 20 seconds or longer, or (2) lasting at least the duration of two missed breaths as determined by baseline breathing pattern, *and* associated with an arousal, an awakening or a ≥3% desaturation. An AHI of >1 event per hour in children is abnormal. An individual sleep specialist can choose to score children ≥13 years using adult criteria.

Central sleep apnea is considered to be due to a loss of ventilatory motor output and may be classified as hypercapnic or normocapnic depending on

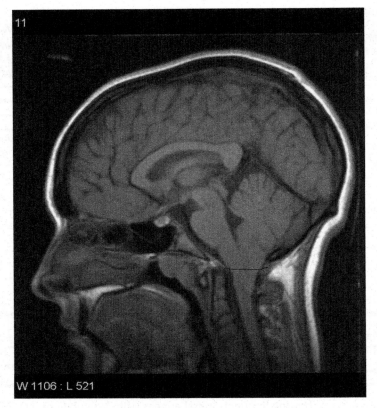

Figure 2.2 Sagittal T1-weighted MRI demonstrating Chiari 1 malformation with low-lying cerebellar tonsils (black horizontal line indicates anatomical threshold).

the level of alveolar hypoventilation. Non-hypercapnic CSA is the most common form and in adults is most often due to congestive heart failure. Central apnea in congestive heart failure is part of periodic breathing or Cheynes–Stokes respiration, with cycles of crescendo–decrescendo breathing with central apnea occurring at the nadir of the ventilatory drive. This condition is rarely seen in childhood. Other etiologies of CSA include periodic breathing at high altitude, hypothyroidism, chronic renal failure, acromegaly and idiopathic CSA when no underlying cause is determined.

Hypercapnic central apnea may be associated with neuromuscular disorders such as muscular dystrophy, amyotrophic lateral sclerosis or kyphoscoliosis. Central congenital hypoventilation syndrome (formerly known as Ondine's curse) is a condition usually diagnosed in infancy and characterized by severe hypoventilation during sleep, with attenuated or absent ventilatory responses to hypercarbia or hypoxia, and associated with autonomic dysfunction. It is caused by a *de novo* mutation in the PHOX2B gene. Chiari malformations have also been reported as causes of central apnea in children, and both normocapnic and hypercapnic patients have been described.

None of the medical etiologies was considered likely in this patient, leading to performance of a cranial MRI. Chiari 1 malformation is a congenital abnormality characterized by caudal herniation of the cerebellar tonsils through the foramen magnum, with resultant crowding at the cranio-cervical junction. It is generally asymptomatic in childhood, and more often is diagnosed in young adults with various symptoms including headache, neck pain, sensory deficits, weakness and occasional cranial nerve or cerebellar dysfunction. With the advent of MRI, asymptomatic Chiari malformations have been identified more frequently and often pose a management dilemma if the symptoms are mild, such as isolated headache. Sleep-disordered breathing, most commonly CSA, has been reported in adults and children with Chiari 1 malformation. The postulated mechanism involves compression or ischemia of the brainstem respiratory centers, dysfunction of the ascending medullary reticular activating system, abnormal ventilatory chemosensitivity and paralysis of movement of the pharyngeal musculature. While CSA has been most commonly reported with Chiari 1 malformations, there are also reports of patients with obstructive or mixed apnea as the predominant presenting symptom, with improvement in sleep-disordered breathing after treatment. Treatment of Chiari 1 malformation involves suboccipital decompression (posterior fossa craniectomy), with or without upper cervical laminectomy. There have been reports of recurrent sleep-disordered breathing after decompressive surgery, presumably due to intrinsic dysfunction of brainstem respiratory centers. Patients should therefore be followed to ensure symptoms do not recur.

Pearls and gold

Central sleep apnea in children is defined as a sleep-related respiratory event associated with absent inspiratory effort throughout the entire duration of the event, lasting 20 seconds or longer or lasting at least the duration of two missed breaths, and associated with an arousal, an awakening or a $\geq 3\%$ desaturation.

Sleep-disordered breathing, most commonly CSA, has been reported in adults and children with Chiari 1 malformation.

Sleep-disordered breathing may recur after decompressive surgery, presumably due to intrinsic dysfunction of brainstem respiratory centers.

SUGGESTED READING

REVIEW

Eckert DJ, Malhotra A, Jordan AS. Mechanisms of apnea. *Prog Cardiovasc Dis* 2009; **51**: 313–23.

GENERAL

Badr MS. Central sleep apnea. *Prim Care Clin Office Pract* 2005; **32**: 361–74.

Dauvilliers Y, Stal V, Abril B, *et al.* Chiari malformation and sleep related breathing disorders. *J Neurol Neurosurg Psychiatry* 2007; **78**: 1344–8.

Murray C, Seton C, Prelog K, Fitzgerald DA. Arnold Chiari type I malformation presenting with sleep disordered breathing in well children. *Arch Dis Child* 2006; **91**: 342–3.

Yglesias A, Narbona J, Vanaclocha V, Artieda J. Chiari type I malformation, glossopharyngeal neuralgia and central sleep apnea in a child. *Dev Med Child Neurol* 1996; **38**: 1126–30.

Case 3

A harsh noise in the night

Giovanna Calandra-Buonaura, Federica Provini
and Pietro Cortelli

Clinical history

Ms. M. consulted a neurologist for the first time at the age of 54 years for a disturbing respiratory noise she presented only during nocturnal sleep. Her husband reported that the noise had probably started 1 year before but its length and intensity had gradually increased, becoming continuous throughout the night. The noise consisted of a strange, high-pitched sound like the bray of a donkey. Sometimes irregular breathing in the form of deep involuntary inspiratory sighs was also present. Ms. M. was unaware of the nocturnal noise and denied abrupt awakenings during the night due to breathing arrest, but complained of diurnal drowsiness and sudden sleep attacks during monotonous activities since the noise started. Deep inspiratory sighs sometimes also occurred during the day when Ms. M. was awake, either at rest or during efforts.

Her husband also described episodes during which Ms. M. seemed to react with sudden violent motor behaviors to something dangerous occurring while she was sleeping, as if she were enacting a dream. During some of the episodes, she had unintentionally injured her husband. The episodes had started 2 years before (at the age of 52) with a high frequency (two to three episodes per night, several nights per week), but had progressively subsided. Ms. M. was again unaware of these episodes and failed to recall any dream with unpleasant or fearful content when she awoke in the morning.

Over the last 2 years, Ms. M. had complained of urinary frequency, urgency and sometimes incontinence. The urinary symptoms were ascribed to bladder prolapse diagnosed after a gynecological examination. When questioned about other symptoms of autonomic dysfunction, Ms. M. also referred to constipation and decreased perspiration.

Ms. M. had suffered an anxious–depressive disorder when she was 25. Her remaining personal history was unremarkable, as was her family history, which was negative for neurological and sleep disorders.

Case Studies in Sleep Neurology: Common and Uncommon Presentations, ed. A. Culebras. Published by Cambridge University Press. © Cambridge University Press 2010.

Examination

General medical and neurological examinations disclosed orthostatic hypotension with a 30 mmHg decrease in systolic blood pressure within 3 minutes of standing from the recumbent position. Her BMI was normal (23 kg/m^2). Cardiovascular responses (systolic and diastolic blood pressure and heart rate) to a 10-minute head-up tilt test at 65° and to the Valsalva maneuver were impaired and consistent with autonomic failure of central origin. Cardiac diseases were excluded by clinical examination and appropriate investigations. Clinical respiratory examination, spirometry, blood gas analysis, and chest and neck CT were normal. Involuntary deep inspiratory sighs (gasps) were occasionally observed while the patient was awake and were not related to a specific effort.

Special studies

The neurologist ordered full-night video-polysomnography (PSG) including electroencephalogram (C3-A2, O2-A1), right and left electro-oculogram, surface EMG of the mylohyoideus, intercostalis, right and left tibialis anterior and extensor carpi radialis muscles, tracheal microphone, oro-nasal airflow, thoracic and abdominal respirograms (strain gauge), ECG, arterial blood pressure (Finapres) and oxyhemoglobin saturation by means of ear oxymeter.

Finally, the neurologist recommended an MRI of the head.

Question

What is your diagnosis? Obstructive sleep apnea syndrome (OSAS)? Catathrenia? Nocturnal stridor? Nocturnal manifestations of broncho-pulmonary disease?

Results of studies

During video-PSG, a harsh, strained, high-pitch inspiratory sound was recorded. The noise was present throughout all sleep phases, but was more pronounced during NREM sleep. It was associated with mild oxyhemoglobin desaturation (between 93 and 90%). Occasional obstructive apneas–hypopneas (apnea–hypopnea index [AHI] <5 per hour), only in the supine position, were also observed. Video-PSG additionally documented a reduction in nocturnal sleep efficiency (81%; normal value: >85%) due to frequent awakenings and a prevalence of light sleep. REM sleep was characterized by abnormal persistence of tonic muscular activity and by increased phasic muscular activity. Episodes of complex vigorous motor behavior were not recorded.

EMG investigation of laryngeal muscle activity was subsequently performed during wakefulness and sleep, placing fine-wire electrodes in the posterior cricoarytenoid, cricothyroid and thyroarytenoid muscles. Vocal cord motion was simultaneously observed with fiberoptic laryngoscopy. Endoesophageal pressure was also recorded using an esophageal balloon. Laryngoscopic investigation showed normal vocal cord motion while Ms. M. was awake and the EMG study failed to disclose signs of neurogenic degeneration in any of the laryngeal muscles examined. The motor pattern of laryngeal muscles was normal during wakefulness, but during sleep, mainly NREM sleep, laryngoscopy showed severe limitation of vocal cord abduction and persistent tonic activity of the adductor laryngeal muscles. The excessive cord adduction and the resulting narrowing of the glottic rimae were responsible for the harsh, strained inspiratory sound recorded during sleep. Endoesophageal pressure showed a wide, increased swing between inspiration and expiration effort associated with stridor (Figure 3.1).

Brain MRI excluded expansive lesions and vascular injury involving the brainstem nuclei implicated in the respiratory and motor control during sleep.

Diagnosis

The specialist made a diagnosis of nocturnal inspiratory "stridor" based on the characteristics of the noise present only during sleep, particularly during NREM sleep. The noise appeared during inspiration, with a higher pitch, associated with only a mild degree of oxyhemoglobin desaturation. The laryngoscopic and EMG patterns observed during sleep documented laryngeal narrowing due to dystonic motion of the vocal cord assumed to be the cause of stridor.

By contrast, narrowing or occlusion of the upper airways at several levels in the pharynx is the cause of snoring and obstructive sleep apneas, which the patient presented only occasionally. Catathrenia, characterized by monotonous and prolonged expiratory groans, occurring during all sleep phases but mainly during REM sleep, was also excluded. Chest and neck masses causing recurrent laryngeal nerve compression or upper-airway obstruction were excluded by a CT scan. Finally, chronic obstructive pulmonary diseases and asthma were excluded by spirometry and blood gas analysis.

A diagnosis of REM-sleep behavior disorder (RBD) was also made due to the characteristic clinical history of violent motor behaviors during sleep associated with PSG evidence of REM sleep without atonia.

General remarks

At the follow-up visit, the specialist gave the results of the investigations to Ms. M. and her husband. He explained that the nocturnal respiratory and

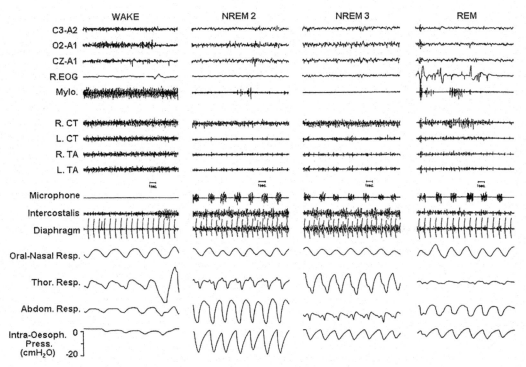

Figure 3.1 Polygraphic recording during electromyographic investigation of the laryngeal muscles disclosed inspiratory stridor (microphone) during all sleep phases and the abnormal persistence of tonic activity on the right cricothyroid muscle. Continuous tonic activity of intercostalis and diaphragmatic muscles during both inspiration and expiration associated with a large and increased swing of endoesophageal pressure were also observed. EEG (C3-A2, O2-A1, CZ-A1); EOG, electro-oculogram; Mylo., mylohyoideus muscle; R., right; L., left; CT, cricothyroid muscle; TA, thyroarytenoid muscle; Oral-Nasal resp., oral–nasal respirogram; Thor. Resp., thoracic respirogram; Abdom. Resp., abdominal respirogram; Intra-Oesoph. Press., endoesophageal pressure.

motor disorders observed (stridor and RBD) and the deep inspiratory sighs (gasps) during wakefulness were probably manifestations of the same disease. Further neurological visits were scheduled every 3–6 months to evaluate the evolution of these disorders and the development of any other neurological symptoms.

In the ensuing 6 years, Ms. M. developed gait ataxia, ocular nystagmus and parkinsonian signs (cogwheel rigidity in the upper and lower limbs and bradykinesia) poorly responsive to levodopa therapy. Orthostatic hypotension progressively increased and became symptomatic, requiring therapy. Finally, stridor worsened, appearing also during wakefulness. Two years after the video-PSG, a new otorhinolaryngological evaluation recommended tracheostomy due to the rapid evolution of the respiratory disorder and the severe limitation of vocal cord abduction occurring during wakefulness.

The neurologist then made a diagnosis of multiple-system atrophy (MSA) based on the presence of autonomic, parkinsonian and cerebellar manifestations and typical sleep disturbances (stridor and RBD). He explained the characteristics of the disease and the therapeutic options used to treat the symptoms to Ms. M. and her husband. He also communicated to Ms. M. and her husband that the prognosis of the disease is unfortunately poor, with a mean survival of about 8–10 years from onset.

Stridor is defined as a harsh, strained high-pitched inspiratory sound, usually described by the bed partner as the bray of a donkey. Stridor in children is frequently a symptom of airway obstruction, mainly due to congenital laryngeal or tracheal anomalies. Psychogenic stridor has also been described in teenage patients. In adulthood, in the absence of anatomic causes of upper-airway obstruction (compressive masses of the neck and thorax), a neurodegenerative disease should be suspected. Multiple-system atrophy is a sporadic adult-onset neurodegenerative disorder characterized by a combination of Parkinsonism, cerebellar features and autonomic failure. Stridor may occur in all clinical stages of MSA, occasionally being the initial symptom of the disease. It is usually present during sleep (nocturnal stridor) together with other sleep-related breathing disorders, namely OSAS and various sleep-related motor disturbances (such as RBD). The frequency of stridor in MSA patients ranges from 13 to 69%; OSAS is also common (from 15 to 37%) and may occur even in the absence of stridor.

Stridor in MSA was initially attributed to denervation of the laryngeal abductor muscles with consequent muscular atrophy and palsy. However, EMG studies have suggested that stridor is determined by sustained tonic activity, such as dystonia, in adductor vocal cord muscles during inspiration causing laryngeal narrowing and airflow limitation. Stridor is also associated with shorter survival and an increased risk of sudden death, presumably due to laryngeal obstruction. Tracheostomy is considered the optimal treatment to prevent sudden death in MSA patients with stridor, but sudden death may occur despite surgery. Continuous positive airway pressure (CPAP) has proved effective in suppressing both stridor and sleep apneas, but it does not always prevent death. In addition, the severity of motor impairment in MSA patients is a limitation for CPAP use.

Pearls and gold

Stridor is defined as a harsh, strained, high-pitched inspiratory sound, usually described by the bed partner as the bray of a donkey.

In adulthood, in the absence of anatomic causes of upper-airway obstruction, a neurodegenerative disease should be suspected.

Stridor may occur in all clinical stages of MSA, occasionally being the initial symptom of the disease.

Stridor is associated with shorter survival and an increased risk of sudden death, presumably due to laryngeal obstruction.

Tracheostomy and CPAP are effective treatments of stridor; however, they do not always prevent death in multiple-system atrophy.

SUGGESTED READING

HISTORICAL

Bannister R, Gibson W, Michaels L, Oppenheimer DR. Laryngeal abductor paralysis in multiple system atrophy. A report on three necropsied cases, with observations on the laryngeal muscles and the nuclei ambigui. *Brain* 1981; **104**: 351–68.

REVIEW

Silber MH, Levine S. Stridor and death in multiple system atrophy. *Mov Disord* 2000; **158**: 699–704.

GENERAL

Gilman S, Wenning GK, Low PA, *et al.* Second consensus statement on the diagnosis of multiple system atrophy. *Neurology* 2008; **71**: 670–6.

Holinger LD. Etiology of stridor in the neonate, infant and child. *Ann Otol Rhinol Laryngol* 1980; **89**: 397–400.

Iranzo A, Santamaría J, Tolosa E, *et al.* Long-term effect of CPAP in the treatment of nocturnal stridor in multiple system atrophy. *Neurology* 2004; **63**: 930–2.

Vetrugno R, Provini F, Cortelli P, *et al.* Sleep disorders in multiple system atrophy: a correlative video-polysomnographic study. *Sleep Med.* 2004; **5**: 21–30.

Vetrugno R, Liguori R, Cortelli P, *et al.* Sleep-related stridor due to dystonic vocal cord motion and neurogenic tachypnea/tachycardia in multiple system atrophy. *Mov Disord* 2007; **22**: 673–8.

Case 4

An infant with obstructed breathing

Zafer N. Soultan and Ran D. Anbar

Clinical history

The patient was a 7.5-month-old Caucasian infant with a birthweight of 3.9 kg, born full term to a 35-year-old mother. The pregnancy was complicated by gestational diabetes. There were no postnatal problems. She developed "noisy breathing" at 1 month of age. During wakefulness, the noise appeared to arise as a result of nasal congestion. During sleep, the noise was reported to sound like snoring. The mother did not observe apnea or disturbed breathing while the patient was asleep.

The patient's pediatrician suspected an upper respiratory tract infection and treated her with "Infants' Cold Formula" with no relief. She was referred to an otolaryngologist, and a soft-tissue X-ray of her neck revealed hypertrophy of her adenoids, which were obstructing the nasal airway.

She underwent an adenoidectomy when she was 6 months old. Post-operatively, while she was asleep in room air, she was observed by the house staff to experience dips in her hemoglobin O_2 saturations to a nadir of 79%. They noted "mild" snoring and paradoxical respiratory efforts, but no apnea.

As no apnea and loud snoring were observed, and as the patient had already undergone an adenoidectomy, sleep-disordered breathing was not considered further at that time. Post-adenoidectomy pulmonary edema was suspected, but her chest X-ray was normal. A cardiovascular anomaly was considered, but a cardiac echo revealed a normal anatomy and no pulmonary hypertension. Her ECG revealed mild right ventricular hypertrophy for age. She underwent a chest CT scan to evaluate for interstitial lung disease, and this study was normal. A 24-hour pH probe study did not demonstrate significant gastroesophageal reflux disease.

Supplemental O_2 via a nasal cannula at 1/8 liter per minute was sufficient to keep her saturation in the high 90s while asleep. She was discharged with home

Case Studies in Sleep Neurology: Common and Uncommon Presentations, ed. A. Culebras. Published by Cambridge University Press. © Cambridge University Press 2010.

pulse oximeter monitoring and O_2 supplementation, and was referred to the Pediatric Apnea and Pulmonary Center.

She was 6.5 months old when she presented for evaluation at our Pediatric Pulmonary Clinic. The mother reported dips in her O_2 saturation to 85% while asleep unless supplemental O_2 was provided. She also described that the patient continued to have "abnormal breath sounds" while asleep and occasional tachypnea. The patient breast-fed with vigor and with no choking, regurgitation or vomiting. She had no history of coughing or wheezing. She had a good weight gain and had attained her developmental milestones appropriately. Her family history was not contributory.

Examination

The physical examination revealed an apparently healthy and well-developed but overweight infant. Her weight was at the 50th percentile for her age, while her height was at the 5th percentile. She did not have craniofacial anomalies. She was breathing through her nose while awake. She had +2 tonsillar hypertrophy. Her lungs were clear. She had normal S_1 and S_2 heart sounds. She had no cardiac murmur. She had normal muscle tone.

On the basis of the history of snoring and paradoxical breathing, and desaturation during sleep, sleep-disordered breathing was suspected and the patient was referred for confirmation by polysomnography (PSG).

Special studies

The PSG was performed when the infant was 7.5 months old. Recorded parameters included an EEG, submental and anterior tibialis EMG, ECG, electro-oculogram (right and left), arterial oxyhemoglobin saturation (SpO$_2$) by pulse oximetry, end-tidal CO_2 (PET$_{CO2}$), oral airflow via thermister, thoracic and abdominal motion by respiratory inductance plethysmography, and a digital video and audio recording.

Question

What is your diagnosis?

Results of studies

The polysomnogram revealed a total sleep time of 408 minutes. Sleep stage distribution was normal. Sleep efficiency was decreased as a result of many arousals and awakenings that were associated with respiratory disturbances.

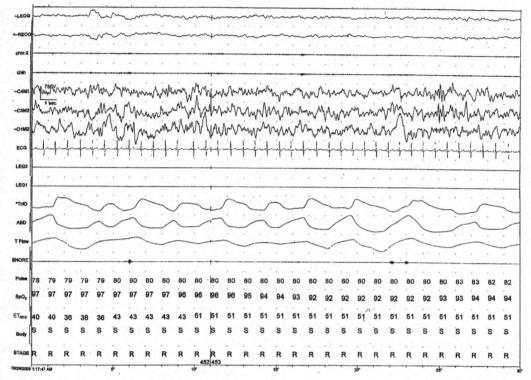

Figure 4.1 This 30-second epoch is from the R stage of this infant's sleep. Note the continuous airflow and respiratory efforts. However, hypoventilation is evident by the paradoxical thoracic/abdominal movements and the development of elevated end-tidal CO_2 (ET_{CO2}) and O_2 desaturation. LEOG/REOG, left/right electro-oculogram; THO, thorax; ABD, abdomen; SpO_2, arterial oxyhemoglobin saturation.

A disturbed breathing pattern was noted. There was mild snoring. There was paradoxical inward rib-cage motion during inspiration throughout much of the study (Figure 4.1). Tachypnea was present, particularly during REM sleep.

There were many central apneas, several obstructive apneas and many hypopneas, some of which were long in duration (Table 4.1). These occurred primarily during REM sleep. Most were associated with hemoglobin desaturations.

Oxygen saturation was 97% during wakefulness. There were many episodes of desaturation. Most episodes of desaturation were moderate, but few were severe. Desaturation episodes occurred primarily during REM sleep. Obstructive apnea episodes were associated with severe desaturation (to a nadir of 65%), but the majority occurred during paradoxical respiration in REM sleep (with a nadir in the mid-80s) (Figure 4.1). There was persistent desaturation during much of REM sleep during obstructive events and a low baseline during prolonged periods

Table 4.1 Breakdown of apnea indexes

	Obstructive apnea	Hypopnea	Mixed apnea	Apnea and hypopnea	Central apnea	Total events
Number of events	12	30	0	42	16	58
Index (episode per hour of sleep)	1.8	4.4	0	6.2	2.4	8.5

of partial obstructive breathing. Her O_2 saturation while she breathed supplemental O_2 at 1/8 liter per minute was normal.

End-tidal CO_2 measurements were normal during wakefulness. Baseline PET_{CO2} measurements during sleep were normal. There were several periods of hypercapnia, but most were mild (mid to high 50s mmHg), occurred during REM sleep and were associated with obstructive apnea or paradoxical breathing (Figure 4.1). As the work of breathing improved after the addition of supplemental O_2, PET_{CO2} improved into the low 50s mmHg.

In summary, this infant had "few" episodes of complete obstruction (apnea) associated with desaturation, and had prolonged periods of partial obstructive breathing (hypoventilation) associated with impairment in gas exchange, which occurred primarily during REM sleep. The respiratory disturbance led to sleep fragmentation.

Diagnosis

The diagnosis based on the PSG results was severe obstructive sleep apnea, pediatric.

Follow-up

The patient was referred to an otolaryngologist. Both residual adenoidal and tonsillar hypertrophy were deemed to be the cause of the sleep-disordered breathing. Revision of the adenoidectomy and tonsillectomy were done. The patient's symptoms and O_2 saturation improved immediately thereafter. A follow-up sleep study 2 months later revealed that the patient no longer demonstrated an obstructive breathing pattern or impairment in gas exchange.

General remarks

Obstructive sleep apnea (OSA) in infants and young children has unique features. This case highlights some of the unique features of obstructive sleep apnea syndrome (OSAS) in infants and young children. Obstructive sleep apnea syndrome is a sleep-related disruption of the normal ventilation and sleep pattern, which results from partial and/or complete upper-airway obstruction. Continuous partial upper-airway obstruction with hypoventilation, as occurred in this case, is more common in infants and young children than complete upper-airway obstruction and apnea.

The effect of upper-airway obstruction on ventilation is more pronounced during REM sleep, because of associated muscle hypotonia. Hypotonia can exacerbate OSA by two mechanisms: (1) it can lead to decreased functional residual capacity, which allows hypoxemia to develop more easily, because there is less O_2 reserve in the lungs when the obstruction occurs; and (2) hypotonia makes it more likely that airway obstruction will develop because the airway is more collapsible. Infants are more affected by OSAS because their chest wall and upper-airway muscles are more compliant than in an older child. Hence, they are prone to a further decline in functional residual capacity and airway obstruction. Additionally, infants spend more time sleeping and more time in REM sleep. Therefore, hypoxemia and hypercapnia can develop more rapidly as a result of partial or complete airway obstruction in infants.

In adults, obstructive events are usually terminated by arousals or awakenings, with subsequent sleep fragmentation, daytime hypersomnolence and poor vigilance. In contrast, arousals are less frequent in infants and children, who are more likely to manifest prolonged episodes of partial obstruction and hypoventilation without an interruption in sleep. Perhaps this is the reason that hypersomnolence is not commonly seen in children.

The leading predisposing factor for OSAS in children is adenotonsillar hypertrophy. Other etiologies include congenital anomalies, especially those involving midfacial hypoplasia or a small nasopharynx or micrognathia, obesity, laryngomalacia and neuromuscular disorders involving muscular hypotonia or hypertonia. In contrast, OSA in adults occurs most commonly as a result of obesity.

The clinical manifestations of OSAS in older children include continuous snoring, difficulty breathing while asleep and restless sleep. Parents are usually concerned and report loud snoring and retractions. Also, parents sometimes describe episodes of increased respiratory efforts with no airflow, followed by gasping, choking, movement or arousal. Children may assume abnormal positions during sleep in order to keep their airway open, e.g. through hyperextension of the neck. Nocturnal enuresis may develop as a result of OSAS in children. Infants' breathing during sleep is shallow and their efforts during obstructive breathing are less forceful than in older children. As they may have little or no snoring, OSAS in infants may be difficult to recognize. It should be suspected in children who are mouth breathers or who have behavioral or learning problems. Infants may have failure to thrive as a consequence of poor feeding and increased work of breathing.

Polysomnography is needed to make the diagnosis of OSAS and differentiate it from primary snoring without airway obstruction. Partial airway obstruction leads to prolonged or continuous periods of hypoventilation, or hypopnea. Periods of obstructive hypoventilation manifest by continuous airflow with snoring, paradoxical breathing, elevated PCO_2 and/or desaturation, and frequent arousals. These periods may not have discrete and identifiable points of start or termination. Therefore, it is essential to monitor for snoring, paradoxical inward-rib-cage motion during inspiration, PET_{CO2} or transcutaneous CO_2 (Ptc_{CO2}), and pulse oximetry in pediatric PSG.

Hypopnea is defined as discrete episodes with a 50% or greater fall in the nasal/oral airflow accompanied by hypoxemia or arousal. Hypopnea in children is scored when it lasts for at least two missed breaths and is associated with arousal, awakening or a decline in saturation of $\geq 3\%$.

Discrete episodes of obstructive apnea may occur in children with OSAS. Studies have found that healthy children exhibit less than one episode of obstructive apnea per hour of sleep. Therefore, an apnea index (AI) of one or more episodes per hour is considered abnormal in children.

In this case, the infant AI was elevated for age, but the pattern of severe obstructive hypoventilation was predominant. This pattern of obstructive hypoventilation is sufficient to diagnose OSAS in children, even without the presence of apnea.

Pearls and gold

OSAS in children is a unique entity and differs significantly from that in adults.

In infants with OSAS, the symptoms may be subtle. It should be suspected in infants with noisy and disturbed breathing during sleep, in particular when associated with desaturation.

The predominant pattern of abnormal breathing in infants and young children with OSAS is persistent partial airway obstruction with hypoventilation during sleep, rather than discrete episodes of obstructive apnea.

It is essential to monitor PET_{CO2} and/or Ptc_{CO2} in pediatric PSG.

SUGGESTED READING

AASM (American Academy of Sleep Medicine). *Manual for the Scoring of Sleep and Associated Events: Rules, Terminology and Technical Specification.* Westchester, Illinois: American Academy of Sleep Medicine, 2007.

AASM (American Academy of Sleep Medicine). *International Classification of Sleep Disorders*, 2nd edn.: *Diagnostic and Coding Manual*. Westchester, Illinois: American Academy of Sleep Medicine, 2005.

American Thoracic Society. Standards and indications for cardiopulmonary sleep studies in children. *Am J Respir Crit Care Med* 1996; **153**: 866–78.

Guilleminault C, Korobkin R, Winkle R. A review of 50 children with obstructive sleep apnea syndrome. *Lung* 1981; **159**: 275–87.

Rosen CL, Anderea LD, Haddad GG. Adult criteria for obstructive sleep apnea do not identify children with serious obstruction. *Am Rev Respir Dis* 1992; **146**: 1231–4.

Ward SL, Marcus CL. Obstructive sleep apnea in infants and young children. *J Clin Neurophysiol* 1996; **13**: 198–207.

Part II

Hypersomnias of central origin

Case 5

My child falls at school

Tik Dion Fung and Marcel Hungs

Clinical history

An 11-year-old Asian–American girl was referred to the Sleep Center for sleep disturbances, excessive daytime sleepiness (EDS) and paroxysmal weakness. The patient had severe daytime sleepiness with an Epworth Sleepiness Scale score of 17 (see Appendix), and had difficulties keeping up with school and friends in her social life. She fell asleep at any time during the day, especially in monotonous situations.

She went to bed at 10 pm, initiating sleep without difficulty. She shared the room with her parents, her grandmother and her younger brother. She denied hypnagogic hallucinations or an uncomfortable feeling in her legs at sleep onset. She was described by her parents as having restless night sleep with frequent awakenings and tossing and turning. She usually woke up at 1 am, with difficulty returning to sleep. She described frequent nightmares causing awakenings. She sometimes saw things that were not present upon awakening. Upon awakening, sleep paralysis was noted. She was woken up at 7 am in order to go to school.

She fell asleep at school and had difficulty staying awake and following presentations in class. When she laughed, she noticed that her mouth corners dropped. With more pronounced emotions such as significant humor or getting angry or scared, her legs gave way so that she would freeze and occasionally fall. This happened up to six times daily. After an earlier evaluation, she was admitted to a children's hospital. She was thought to have depressive symptoms. She was prescribed amitriptyline up to 125 mg without improvement of her nocturnal and daytime symptoms. Her past medical history and family history was unremarkable. She was referred to a child neurologist who started a work-up for myasthenia gravis and an unsuccessful empiric treatment with acetylcholinesterase inhibitor. Twenty-four-hour EEG monitoring did not demonstrate any ictal events. A brain MRI was normal without any structural lesion, and electrodiagnostic studies were normal without findings for neuropathy, myopathy or myasthenia

Case Studies in Sleep Neurology: Common and Uncommon Presentations, ed. A. Culebras. Published by Cambridge University Press. © Cambridge University Press 2010.

gravis. Laboratory studies were unrevealing (including vitamin B_{12}, folate, iron studies and electrolytes). An evaluation at the sleep center was initiated.

Examination

General and neurological examinations were normal.

Special studies

The patient was asked to keep a 14-day sleep log with event documentation. Nocturnal video-polysomnography (PSG) immediately followed by a multiple sleep latency test (MSLT) were ordered.

Question

Could it be narcolepsy at this early age?

Results of studies

The video-PSG results showed that there were 8 hours and 4 minutes of sleep time. Sleep efficiency was 94%. REM sleep onset was after 36 minutes of sleep. The apnea–hypopnea index (AHI) was 1.2 per hour with mostly obstructive hypopneas. Fragmented night sleep was noted with a spontaneous microarousal index of 13 per hour.

In a five-nap MSLT, mean sleep latency was 0.7 minutes. The sleep latency for the first four naps was 0 minutes. In the last nap, she had a sleep latency of 3.5 minutes. She went into REM sleep immediately, without going into any other sleep stages at the beginning of the MSLT in three of the five naps (Figure 5.1).

Diagnosis

The diagnosis was narcolepsy with cataplexy.

Follow-up

CSF hypocretin analysis was not performed in light of the diagnostic certainty, given her history of EDS with cataplexy, hypnopompic hallucinations and the MSLT results. After the initial sleep clinic consultation, she was started on modafinil 200 mg, with significant improvement of her daytime sleepiness and school performance. Sertraline 50 mg decreased the frequency and severity of

LOC-A2

ROC-A1

C3-A2

C4-A1

O1-A2

O2-A1

CHIN

ECG

CHIN 2

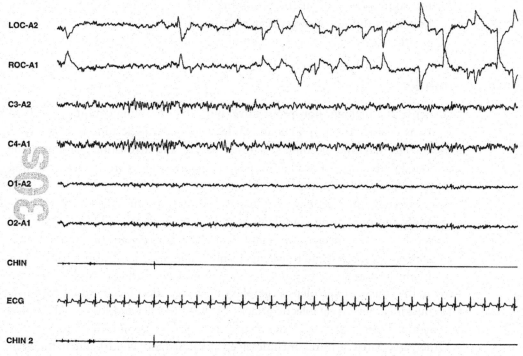

Figure 5.1 Thirty-second epoch showing sleep-onset REM in the first epoch of nap 3 of the MSLT recording. Note the vigorous eye movements in leads LOC-A2 and ROC-A1 and the absence of muscle tone in the chin EMG. LOC, left oculogram; ROC, right oculogram. The EEG leads show low voltage and intermixed activity.

cataplexy. Her daytime sleepiness was significantly reduced. She was able to keep up in school. Her grades improved and she was able to maintain social interaction with friends. Her mother also noted that, although her cataplexy had significantly improved, every day after school, she had "balance problems." She would recover within seconds from her cataplectic events.

In subsequent follow-up visits, sodium oxybate was administered and titrated up to 3 g twice nightly, which helped further decrease her cataplexy to once or twice daily. Her sleep also improved without frequent awakenings. However, at the higher dose of sodium oxybate, she was noted to have frequent nocturnal movements that resembled brief repetitive myoclonic jerking movements by description, and her mother decided to stop the medication.

Without the sodium oxybate, the girl again experienced significant EDS and cataplexy. After counseling of the parents, sodium oxybate was restarted and PSG was repeated on sodium oxybate. Sleep study results revealed a sleep efficiency of 98% with 63% sleep stage N3 and with immediate onset of sleep. The patient took her sodium oxybate at the beginning of the recording as well as at 2 am. The sleep study did not show evidence of clinical ictal events.

The patient now only experiences minimal cataplexy and little or no EDS.

General remarks

Narcolepsy is a lifelong, non-progressive, but often disabling condition of REM sleep. It is characterized by EDS and sudden loss of muscle tone if cataplexy is present. The daytime sleepiness is often severe and irresistible, and may be manifested in the form of sudden sleep attacks. Sleep attacks are an overwhelming urge to sleep within minutes.

Excessive daytime sleepiness is often the first symptom of narcolepsy and is commonly the presenting complaint requiring medical attention. Sleepiness in narcolepsy is often severe, culminating in sudden sleep attacks. Cataplexy is characterized by sudden and transient episodes of loss of muscle tone without loss of consciousness triggered by emotions such as laughter, surprise, anger or humor. Early in the course of narcolepsy, cataplexy may only affect facial muscles or cause knee buckling. Severe cataplectic attacks can lead to falls and loss of all striated muscle tone of the extremities; the events can last from seconds to minutes.

Other associated features include sleep paralysis and vivid hallucinations at sleep onset (hypnagogic) or on awakening (hypnopompic).

In narcolepsy, there is abnormal regulation of the sleep/wake cycle and increased incursion of REM sleep. Pathophysiology is associated with hypocretin/orexin peptides, which are exclusively produced by neurons in the lateral hypothalamus. A putative flip/flop switch has been proposed for control of REM sleep, where hypocretin neurons are hypothesized to excite the "REM-off" neuron population in the mesopontine tegmentum. Most patients with narcolepsy and cataplexy display low or undetectable concentrations of hypocretin in their CSF, and post-mortem binding studies demonstrate a marked decrease in hypocretin-containing neurons in the hypothalamus. An autoimmune cause, with genetic predisposition, is suspected but not proven. Rare cases of secondary narcolepsy have been reported in patients with brain lesions (mostly located in the posterior hypothalamus, midbrain and pons).

Age of onset varies between childhood and middle age, with a large peak at age 15 years and a small peak at 36 years. Daytime sleepiness is usually the first symptom, with onset of cataplexy within 1 year. In younger children, cataplexy and other REM-sleep phenomena can develop with some delay. When cataplexy develops in children, it is often mistaken as epileptic seizures such as atonic seizures, or as weakness caused by neuromuscular disorders. Sleepiness and cataplexy generally persist throughout life.

There are three main types of narcolepsy: narcolepsy with cataplexy, narcolepsy without cataplexy and secondary narcolepsy due to a medical condition. The ICSD-2 (AASM, 2005) diagnostic criteria for narcolepsy require a complaint of EDS occurring almost daily for at least 3 months. A definite history of cataplexy is present in narcolepsy with cataplexy. The diagnosis should, whenever possible, be confirmed by nocturnal PSG followed by MSLT. Polysomnography is performed primarily to exclude other causes of daytime sleepiness such as sleep apnea, and to ensure that patients have at least 6 hours of sleep prior to MSLT on the following day. In narcolepsy with cataplexy, the mean sleep latency on MSLT is less than or equal to 8 minutes, and two or more short-onset REM-sleep periods are observed following sufficient nocturnal sleep (minimum 6 hours). In patients without cataplexy, confirmatory sleep studies are required for diagnosis. Alternatively, a CSF hypocretin concentration of less than 110pg/ml is a highly specific but moderately sensitive criterion in narcolepsy with cataplexy, but not in narcolepsy without cataplexy. There is a strong association with the HLA DQB1*0602 genotype, but this is neither sensitive nor specific in diagnosis. Nonetheless, these ancillary CSF and blood tests may be helpful in cases where the sleep studies are unavailable or non-diagnostic, or when history is difficult to obtain, such as in children. Differential diagnoses to keep in mind are conditions of sleep fragmentation, such as obstructive sleep apnea syndrome (OSAS) and periodic limb movements of sleep (PLMS), idiopathic hypersomnia, recurrent hypersomnia, hypersomnia associated with depression, chronic sleep deprivation, syncope, delayed sleep phase syndrome, metabolic conditions, seizures, attention deficit syndrome and poor sleep hygiene.

As per the most recent practice parameters for the treatment of narcolepsy, the treatment objectives should include control of sleepiness and other sleep-related symptoms when present. Most medications used are off-label in children. Modafinil is effective for the treatment of daytime sleepiness due to narcolepsy in children (although modafinil is not FDA approved for patients under 18 years). It has emerged as the first-line treatment for most patients. Recently, armodafinil at a dose of 150 or 250mg daily was approved to treat narcolepsy in adults. Sodium oxybate is effective for treatment of narcolepsy and cataplexy, daytime sleepiness and disrupted sleep at a dose of 4.5g twice a night. It is the only drug that can alleviate all the core symptoms of narcolepsy. Its prescription is highly regulated in Europe and the USA due to its potential non-medical use as a mind-altering drug. Amphetamine, methamphetamine, dextroamphetamine and methylphenidate are effective for treatment of daytime sleepiness due to narcolepsy and have a long history of effective use in clinical practice, but there is limited information available on the benefit-to-risk ratio in children. Scheduled naps can be beneficial to combat sleepiness but seldom suffice as the primary therapy for narcolepsy. Tricyclic antidepressants, selective serotonin reuptake inhibitors (SSRIs) and venlafaxine may be effective treatment for cataplexy.

The experience of children with narcolepsy and cataplexy is one of significant psychosocial impairment across interpersonal, vocational, educational and family life. Significant levels of stigma associated with the illness can lead to a sense of shame, reactive depression and isolation. Strategies to facilitate the well-being of children with narcolepsy must include the improvement of EDS and REM-sleep-related phenomena, as well as addressing psychological stressors and potentially long-term disabilities. The ultimate goal in the treatment of narcolepsy with cataplexy remains a normal life with an unobstructed path, meeting all personal and academic goals.

Pearls and gold

The experience of children with narcolepsy and cataplexy is one of significant psychosocial impairment across interpersonal, vocational, educational and family life.

When cataplexy develops in children, it is often mistaken as epileptic seizures such as atonic seizures, or as weakness caused by neuromuscular disorders.

Modafinil is effective for the treatment of daytime sleepiness due to narcolepsy in children, although it is not FDA approved for patients under 18 years.

Sodium oxybate is effective for treatment of narcolepsy and cataplexy, daytime sleepiness and disrupted sleep at a dose of 4.5g twice a night, but its prescription is highly regulated due to its potential non-medical use as a mind-altering drug.

SUGGESTED READING

AASM (American Academy of Sleep Medicine). *International Classification of Sleep Disorders*, 2nd edn.: *Diagnostic and Coding Manual*. Westchester, Illinois: American Academy of Sleep Medicine, 2005.

Hungs M, Mignot E. Hypocretin/orexin, sleep and narcolepsy. *Bioessays* 2001; **23**: 397–408.

Lu J, Sherman D, Devor M, *et al*. A putative flip–flop switch for control of REM sleep. *Nature* 2006; **441**: 589–94.

Morgenthaler TI, Kapur VK, Brown T, *et al*. Standards of Practice Committee of the American Academy of Sleep Medicine. Practice parameters for the treatment of narcolepsy and other hypersomnias of central origin. *Sleep* 2007; **30**: 1705–11.

Nevsimalova S. Narcolepsy in childhood. *Sleep Med Rev* 2009; **13**: 169–80.

Case 6

A sleepy-head

Antonio Culebras

Clinical history

Mr. X. remembered being a sleepy-head in high school. He would sleep through study hall and had great difficulty staying awake in morning classes. College had been a struggle as well. Now, 25 years old and recently married, Mr. X. decided to visit a sleep specialist because of insomnia. He had no difficulty falling asleep, but lately he had had many awakenings through the night that were disturbing his newlywed wife. On several occasions, he had awakened in the middle of the night unable to move or shout, despite a sense of growing fright. The episodes lasted less than a minute and had caused anxiety. On specific questioning, Mr. X. acknowledged falling asleep while driving, only to be awakened by the noise caused when riding over the rumble-strips on the side of the road. He would take naps almost daily that were refreshing and always associated with vivid dreams. He denied episodes of sudden falls, but remembered that, at his wedding ceremony, he had suddenly become unable to stand from a kneeling position and his head keeled over as if in deep prayer, an action that witnesses attributed to the intensity of the moment.

Examination

The neurology specialist in sleep disorders evaluating Mr. X. elicited a normal neurological examination.

Special studies

The specialist ordered nocturnal polysomnography (PSG), followed by a multiple sleep latency test (MSLT).

Case Studies in Sleep Neurology: Common and Uncommon Presentations, ed. A. Culebras. Published by Cambridge University Press. © Cambridge University Press 2010.

Question

What is your diagnosis: insomnia or hypersomnia?

Follow-up

The specialist advised Mr. X. not to drive unless accompanied and only during daytime hours, as well as to avoid driving for more than 30 minutes or on long stretches of road. He also recommended 20-minute naps after lunch and when returning home from work. Medication would not be prescribed until the results of the sleep study became available.

Results of studies

Two weeks later, the sleep study showed a nocturnal short-onset REM sleep latency of 7.5 minutes. The proportion of nocturnal REM sleep was 27%, which was high for the standards of the laboratory. Sleep apnea and periodic limb movements were not found. The MSLT showed the presence of REM sleep in all four naps with a latency of 5 minutes. Average sleep latency was 2 minutes.

Diagnosis

Given these results, the specialist made a diagnosis of narcolepsy with possible cataplexy and decided not to pursue a CSF hypocretin analysis in light of the diagnostic certainty of the PSG results.

General remarks

At the follow-up visit, the specialist gave Mr. X. and his wife an overview of the test results, prognosis of the disorder and management. He prescribed modafinil 200 mg to be taken in the morning, a dose that could be increased to 400 mg if necessary. He also prescribed a hypnotic of short duration to take at bedtime and recommended two daily 20-minute naps. Once again, he counseled the patient not to drive under certain conditions and gave him brochures with additional information on narcolepsy, as well as the addresses of various narcolepsy organizations and support groups. A second follow-up visit was scheduled for 3 months later to review the efficacy of the medication and consider other pharmacological alternatives, if warranted. The patient was advised that another new medication, armodafinil, had recently become available and was prescribed at doses of 150–250 mg daily.

Narcolepsy is a life-long disorder presenting with excessive daytime sleepiness (EDS) and, ironically, with fragmented sleep that may lead to an erroneous diagnosis of insomnia. Cataplexy, or sudden loss of muscle tone, may or may not occur. Additional manifestations are sleep paralysis and vivid dreams at sleep onset, also called hypnagogic hallucinations. Most cases of narcolepsy with cataplexy are associated with the loss of approximately 50,000–100,000 hypothalamic neurons containing hypocretin. In patients with bona fide narcolepsy, CSF analysis shows levels of hypocretin below 110 pg/ml. Symptomatic narcolepsy, also known as narcolepsy due to medical condition, refers to conditions resembling narcolepsy that have a well-defined etiology or are associated with known co-morbidity, generally a structural lesion involving the diencephalic region.

In addition to modafinil, patients may respond favorably to the administration of methylphenidate and dexedrine. Cataplexy responds to the administration of imipramine, clomipramine, protriptyline and fluoxetine. Sodium oxybate is FDA approved and is the drug of choice for patients with narcolepsy/cataplexy who have not responded to other measures, particularly if the triad of excessive sleepiness, cataplexy and nocturnal sleep disruption is present.

Pearls and gold

Narcolepsy is a life-long disorder presenting with EDS, sometimes with cataplexy, and, ironically, with fragmented sleep, which may lead to an erroneous diagnosis of insomnia.

Most cases of narcolepsy with cataplexy are associated with the loss of approximately 50,000–100,000 hypothalamic neurons containing hypocretin.

CSF analysis shows levels of hypocretin below 110 pg/ml.

Sodium oxybate is FDA approved and is the drug of choice for patients with narcolepsy/cataplexy who have not responded to other measures, particularly if the triad of excessive sleepiness, cataplexy and nocturnal sleep disruption is present.

SUGGESTED READING

HISTORICAL

Passouant P. The history of narcolepsy. In: Guilleminault C, Dement WC, Passouant P, eds. *Narcolepsy*. New York: Spectrum, 1976; 3–14.

Wilson S. The narcolepsies. *Brain* 1928; **51**: 63–77.

REVIEW

Baumann CR, Bassetti CL. Hypocretins (orexins) and sleep-wake disorders. *Lancet Neurol* 2005; **4**: 673–82.

GENERAL

AASM (American Academy of Sleep Medicine). *International Classification of Sleep Disorders*, 2nd edn.: *Diagnostic and Coding Manual.* Westchester, Illinois: American Academy of Sleep Medicine, 2005.

Littner MR, Kushida C, Wise M, *et al.* Practice parameters for clinical use of the multiple sleep latency test and the maintenance of wakefulness test. *Sleep* 2005; **28**: 113–21.

Mignot E, Lammers GJ, Ripley B, *et al.* The role of cerebrospinal fluid hypocretin measurement in the diagnosis of narcolepsy and other hypersomnias. *Arch Neurol* 2002; **59**: 1553–62.

Morgenthaler TI, Kapur VK, Brown T, *et al.* Standards of Practice Committee of the American Academy of Sleep Medicine. Practice parameters for the treatment of narcolepsy and other hypersomnias of central origin. *Sleep* 2007; **30**: 1705–11.

Silber MH, Rye DB. Solving the mystery of narcolepsy. The hypocretin story. *Neurology* 2001; **56**: 1616–18.

Weaver TE, Cuéllar N. A randomized trial evaluating the effectiveness of sodium oxybate therapy on quality of life in narcolepsy. *Sleep* 2006; **29**: 1189–94.

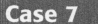

Case 7

A roller-coaster of neurological diagnoses

Baruch El-Ad

Clinical history

AB, a 17-year-old girl, was evaluated for excessive daytime sleepiness (EDS). She was born at term to healthy unrelated parents through cesarean section due to prolonged labor. She suffered developmental delay, and was later diagnosed with mild mental retardation (IQ 70). No further details about the specific diagnosis were available. She studied in a special education system.

At the age of 4 years, she started to fall asleep and become unresponsive for several minutes, sometimes several times a day. Repeated EEG studies were reported normal. A brain MRI was normal. She was diagnosed with atonic seizures and treated with valproate. Her parents thought that the episodes were less frequent with valproate, so she remained under the care of a community neurologist and was not referred to a specialty center. She became increasingly sleepy during the day and the sleepiness was attributed to a side effect of valproate. She had to take naps during daytime hours. On one occasion, she awakened from a nap and was unable to move or talk for about 4 hours, but was able to move her eyes in all directions. Following this episode, she was admitted for evaluation to the Department of Neurology. During the admission, the patient had multiple episodes of non-responsiveness lasting minutes to hours; at this time, her EEG showed normal wakefulness and non-specific generalized dysrhythmia.

Examination

Her height was 161 cm and weight was 60 kg; the patient was fully cooperative. The neurological examination was within normal limits. During one of the prolonged (about 10 minutes) periods of non-responsiveness, the patient lay with her eyes shut, there were rapid eye movements behind closed eyelids and she had flaccid or fluctuating muscle tone, and was non-responsive to verbal or painful stimuli; she later had an almost full recall for test sentences asked during this period.

Case Studies in Sleep Neurology: Common and Uncommon Presentations, ed. A. Culebras. Published by Cambridge University Press. © Cambridge University Press 2010.

Special studies

Nocturnal polysomnography (PSG) and a multiple sleep latency test (MSLT) were carried out.

Question

What is your working diagnosis and how do you account for the prolonged periods of unprovoked non-responsiveness with fluctuating muscle tone?

Results of studies

Nocturnal PSG showed a sleep latency of 15 minutes and REM sleep latency of 10 minutes, and total sleep time was 7 hours, 10 minutes; sleep efficiency was low for age at 82%, with multiple awakenings. The proportion of stage N1 sleep was 14% of total sleep time, stage N2 was 60%, stage N3 was 10% and REM sleep was 16%. There was neither sleep-disordered breathing nor periodic limb movements. A MSLT showed an average sleep latency of 3.6 minutes, with five sleep-onset REM sleep periods.

Diagnosis

The diagnosis was childhood-onset narcolepsy with cataplexy. The parents declined CSF testing for hypocretin.

Follow-up

Valproate was discontinued. The patient was started on methylphenidate 30 mg per day for sleepiness and paroxetine 10 mg per day for cataplexy; the doses were subsequently doubled. The patient responded extremely well: the episodes of cataplexy all but disappeared, and the sleepiness decreased significantly. Her functioning in school and in the community improved significantly. About 1 year later, while on a stable dose of methylphenidate and paroxetine, she was admitted to a psychiatric hospital due to bizarre behavior and multimodal hallucinations. A psychotic disorder was diagnosed.

Follow-up question

Would a psychotic event be related to narcolepsy or the treatment received?

Extended follow-up

Methylphenidate was discontinued and the patient was given modafinil 200 mg per day. She continued to receive paroxetine and was also given risperidone

8 mg per day to control her psychosis; this was later changed to parenteral zuclopenthixol decanoate every 4 weeks as maintenance therapy. Within several months (about 2 years after the diagnosis of narcolepsy), her condition stabilized enough to allow gradual discontinuation of the neuroleptic therapy. She remained on paroxetine and modafinil. Sleepiness was under reasonable control, but she continued to experience cataplexy attacks 10–15 times a month. She gained weight following neuroleptic therapy reaching 84 kg. Sodium oxybate was unavailable at her place of residence, and she received clomipramine 150 mg per day for cataplexy, instead of paroxetine, with somewhat better control of her symptoms. At the age of 19 years, she left home and lived in a hostel with community supervision by certified social workers. She obtained a job in a factory that made cardboard boxes, but she frequently missed work, complaining of "not feeling well." Her personal supervising social worker thought she might not be fully compliant with the medication schedule or that she might be feigning cataplexy attacks for secondary gain.

General remarks

The diagnosis of narcolepsy with cataplexy was sustained over the years. The onset of narcolepsy may occur with any of the four cardinal symptoms (excessive sleepiness, sleep paralysis, hypnagogic hallucinations and cataplexy), the most frequent being EDS. Cataplexy usually follows EDS, and it may appear years later. Cataplexy as the presenting symptom of narcolepsy is relatively uncommon, and occurs in 5–10% of patients; in these cases, atonic epilepsy is in the differential diagnosis (as are other disorders causing rapid development of weakness, e.g. periodic paralyses). In our patient, sleepiness, which followed cataplexy several months later, was erroneously attributed to a side effect of valproate and was not questioned for many years because it was the parents' impression that valproate was somewhat helpful in reducing the atonic "seizures."

Childhood onset of narcolepsy is uncommon, but has been reported. The usual age of onset is mid- to late teens up to mid-20s. Occasionally patients may become ill after the age of 40.

Prolonged periods of non-responsiveness in patients with cataplexy have been dubbed *status cataplecticus*; the muscle tone may wax and wane, and various muscle groups may take part in the process, sometimes producing myoclonus when the tone abruptly returns to previously atonic muscles. *Status cataplecticus* may occur after abrupt withdrawal of medications used to treat cataplexy. The most frequent precipitating factor for cataplexy is strong emotion, but in this patient's case, cataplexy was unusual because it apparently occurred unprovoked and was very prolonged.

Psychosis can be a side effect of stimulants (amphetamines and methylphenidate). Even modafinil, which is generally considered a safer drug, is not devoid of this potentially dangerous side effect. The dose of methylphenidate in this patient (about 1 mg/kg) was not high enough to consider psychosis a side effect 1 year after stabilization of treatment responses; however, given the possibility, it was discontinued. Another vexing problem posed was the potential increase in symptoms of EDS with neuroleptic medications by partially blocking dopaminergic transmission.

Psychosis, even frank schizophrenia, can be a manifestation of narcolepsy. Moreover, narcolepsy may be misdiagnosed as schizophrenia, due to florid multi-modal hallucinations and bizarre behavior, which may at times be so dominant as to obscure other manifestations of narcolepsy, as in our patient's case. It was difficult to determine whether psychosis was co-morbid with narcolepsy or part of the narcolepsy spectrum of symptomatology. The therapeutic dilemma became even more poignant, as an increase in stimulant dosage might be indicated for control of narcolepsy, rather than tapering, should an adverse reaction to treatment be the cause. The psychiatrists treating the patient were not comfortable administering high-dose stimulants to a hallucinating patient and their approach prevailed; the patient received neuroleptic medication and gradually improved.

Feigned cataplectic attacks in patients with cataplexy can happen, as can pseudoseizures in epileptic patients. The psychological mechanisms underlying these spells are unknown, but they undoubtedly complicate the care of patients.

It is known that narcolepsy is associated with excessive weight gain and, over time, our patient became obese. Obesity management may help reduce sleepiness secondary to sleep-disordered breathing and a follow-up polysomnogram might be indicated. Psychosocial support should be provided on a continuous basis.

Pearls and gold

Childhood onset of narcolepsy is uncommon, but has been described.

Cataplexy as the presenting symptom of narcolepsy is relatively uncommon, occurring in 5–10% of all patients. It must be included in the differential diagnosis of atonic seizures, especially before EDS settles in.

Cataplexy may take the form of prolonged waxing and waning, with partial or complete muscle atonia, called *status cataplecticus*.

Psychosis can be a side effect of stimulant administration.

Schizophrenia may be co-morbid or an intrinsic manifestation of narcolepsy.

Obesity is frequently observed in association with narcolepsy, contributing to sleepiness.

SUGGESTED READING

HISTORICAL

Yoss RE, Daly DD. Criteria for the diagnosis of the narcoleptic syndrome. *Mayo Clin Proc* 1957; **32**: 320–8.

REVIEW

Bassetti CL. Narcolepsy. In: Culebras A, ed. *Sleep Disorders and Neurological Diseases*, 2nd edn. New York: Informa Healthcare, 2007; 83–116.

GENERAL

Auger RR, Goodman SH, Silber MH, *et al*. Risks of high dose stimulants in the treatment of disorders of excessive somnolence: a case–control study. *Sleep* 2005; **28**: 667–72.

Douglass AB, Hays P, Pazderka F, Russel JM. Florid refractory schizophrenias that turn out to be treatable variants of HLA-associated narcolepsy. *J Nerv Ment Dis* 1991; **179**: 12–17.

Guilleminault C, Pelayo R. Narcolepsy in prepubertal children. *Ann Neurol* 1998; **43**: 135–42.

Kondziella D, Arlien-Soborg P. Diagnostic and therapeutic challenges in narcolepsy-related psychosis. *J Clin Psychiatry* 2006; **67**: 1817–19.

Krahn LE, Hansen MR, Shepard JW. Pseudocataplexy. *Psychosomatics* 2001; **42**: 356–8.

Parkes JD, Baraitser M, Marsden CD, Asselman P. Natural history, symptoms and treatment of the narcoleptic syndrome. *Acta Neurol Scand* 1975; **52**: 337–53.

Part III

Circadian rhythm disorders

A shift worker falls repeatedly

Teresa Canet

Clinical history

Mr. C. was a 30-year-old man referred by his physician to the sleep disorders clinic complaining of uncontrolled daytime sleepiness and generalized muscle hypotonic attacks. He was falling to the ground without loss of consciousness and the attacks were triggered by laughter. There was a history of sleep paralysis over the past 2 years. Falling happened for the first time while playing tennis, and later when laughing or joking around. In the beginning, only his legs were affected, but more recently all muscles were involved, including the face. Sudden sleep attacks had happened during active work for the past 2 years. In recent months, he had had two car accidents because of falling asleep while driving short distances (5 miles). The symptoms affected the patient's quality of life, having a major impact upon recreation, occupation and work performance.

He was a supervisor in a textile company and worked 12-hour shifts: 2 am to 2 pm or 2 pm to 2 am, sleeping an average of 7.5 hours a day in two discontinuous periods depending on his shifts. When he worked the night shift, he slept from 3 pm to 7 pm and 10 pm to 1 am. On day shifts, he slept from 3 am to 8 am and 11.30 am to 1 pm. He usually slept on his side, snoring occasionally. There was no history of apnea, periodic limb movements (PLMs), somniloquy or bizarre behaviors during sleep.

Cardiorespiratory and neurological examinations were normal. Blood test results and an MRI of the brain were normal.

Special studies

Polysomnography (PSG) was registered at the end of his vacation period. Before PSG, the patient completed a 14-day sleep diary. The average sleep time was 7.30 hours and no deprivation was found. A multiple sleep latency test (MSLT) with four naps at 2-hour intervals followed the nocturnal study.

Case Studies in Sleep Neurology: Common and Uncommon Presentations, ed. A. Culebras. Published by Cambridge University Press. © Cambridge University Press 2010.

Table 8.1 MSLT results

	Nap 1	Nap 2	Nap 3	Nap 4	Average
Lights out	7.58 am	9.50 am	11.51 am	1.48 pm	—
Onset sleep	8.00 am	9.52 am	11.53 am	1.51 pm	—
Lights on	8.19 am	10.07 am	12.08 am	2.05 pm	—
Time in bed (min)	21	17.0	17.0	17	17.8
Total sleep time (min)	20.0	16.0	16.5	15.5	17.0
Sleep latency (min)	1.0	1.5	1.5	2.5	1.6
REM-sleep latency (min)	0.0	0.5	1.5	1.5	0.9

Question

What is the clinical diagnosis: narcolepsy with cataplexy or possible shift work sleep disorder?

Results of studies

Polysomnography showed a total sleep time of 400 minutes (6.7 hours) and a total wake time of 40 minutes. Sleep efficiency was 91%. Latency to sleep onset (stage N1) and stages N2 and N3 were shortened (0.5, 8.5 and 17.5 minutes, respectively). REM-sleep latency was normal (97 minutes). The respiratory disturbance index was normal and PLMs were not observed. The MSLT recording showed that the patient slept in all four naps; mean sleep latency was 1.6 minutes. The presence of REM sleep was recorded in four naps with an average REM-sleep latency of 0.9 minutes (Table 8.1).

Diagnosis

The diagnosis was narcolepsy with cataplexy in a shift worker (classified as hypersomnia of central origin not due to circadian rhythm disorder, sleep-related breathing disorder or other cause of disturbed nocturnal sleep (ICSD-2; AASM, 2005).

Follow-up

Treatment began in September 2003 with clomipramine in increasing daily doses from 25 to 75 mg. Control of cataplexy was not complete but was acceptable (less than one episode per month on average). After a year and half, the frequency of cataplexy attacks increased to four to seven episodes per week, which was interpreted as a phenomenon of tolerance, and clomipramine was replaced with fluoxetine (40 mg per day). Fluoxetine did not control cataplexy satisfactorily and the patient was still reporting an average of 3.4 attacks per week. At this time, the patient completed a sleep diary where he noted sleep/wake schedules and cataplexy and sleep attacks (Figure 8.1). Fluoxetine was withdrawn gradually over a month.

After a 3-week drug washout period, sodium oxybate was administered in increasing doses, initially 4.5 mg per day for 2 weeks and then 6 mg per day, the current dose. The administration of sodium oxybate was determined by work timetables and wake/sleep schedules as follows: 6 mg per day divided into two equal doses. The patient took a first 3 mg dose at bedtime and a second dose about 3 hours later, when he slept for 7 hours continuously or before the second separate sleep period. Progression in a year and a half to 6 mg per day was satisfactory; no episodes of cataplexy occurred during regular work hours or when practicing sports (tennis, jogging and handball). Hypersomnia due to narcolepsy was treated with modafinil and was co-administered with the drugs for cataplexy. He stopped taking modafinil of his own accord after 4 months of treatment with sodium oxybate and does not complain of daytime sleepiness to date. He now reports a continuous sleep pattern without dreams or sleep fragmentation, and wakes up feeling rested and refreshed.

General remarks

Narcolepsy is a chronic sleep disorder. The clinical features are excessive daytime sleepiness (EDS), cataplexy, sleep paralysis, hypnagogic hallucinations, fragmented night-time sleep and automatic behaviors. Cataplexy is the most specific symptom of narcolepsy consisting of an abrupt bilateral loss of skeletal muscle tone. Episodes are triggered most commonly by laughter, but may also be caused by sudden emotional reactions such as anger, surprise or fear. Narcolepsy associated with cataplexy is caused by the selective loss of relatively few neurons responsible for producing hypocretin in the hypothalamus.

Clinical manifestations, PSG and MSLT were used to diagnose the condition, although according to ICSD-1 diagnostic criteria (AASM, 2001), the presence of EDS and cataplexy is sufficient for a definitive diagnosis. The diagnosis should be confirmed with an MSLT (mean sleep latency ≤8 minutes and two or more sleep-onset REM periods), as established by the current international diagnostic criteria (ICSD-2; AASM, 2005). Cataplexy was assessed by simple subjective reporting. Subjective validated scales or questionnaires are also available: the Stanford Cataplexy Questionnaire (Anic-Labat et al., 1999), Ullanlinna Narcolepsy Scale (Hublin et al., 1994) and postural atonia scales (Parkes et al., 1998).

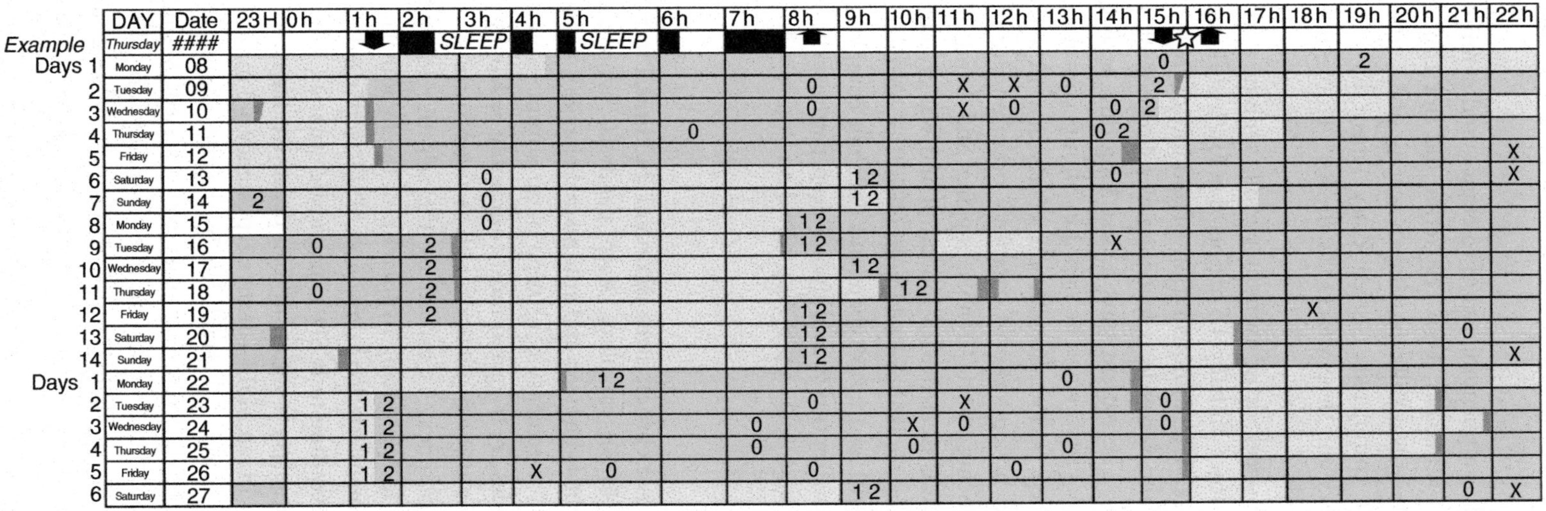

DAY	Date	23H	0h	1h	2h	3h	4h	5h	6h	7h	8h	9h	10h	11h	12h	13h	14h	15h	16h	17h	18h	19h	20h	21h	22h
Example Thursday	###			→	*SLEEP*	*SLEEP*	*SLEEP*											0							
Days 1 Monday	08																	2				2			
2 Tuesday	09										0			X	X	0		2							X
3 Wednesday	10								0		0			X	X		0	0 2							X
4 Thursday	11																0 2	0 2							
5 Friday	12															0									
6 Saturday	13				0						1 2	1 2													
7 Sunday	14	2			0						1 2	1 2													
8 Monday	15				0																				
9 Tuesday	16		0		2											X									
10 Wednesday	17		0		2						1 2	1 2													
11 Thursday	18				2						1 2	1 2	1 2				X			X					
12 Friday	19										1 2				0										
13 Saturday	20							1 2			1 2				0										
14 Sunday	21																							0	
Days 1 Monday	22										0			X	0										X
2 Tuesday	23			1 2						0			X			0		0							
3 Wednesday	24			1 2						0	0		0					0							
4 Thursday	25			1 2							0														
5 Friday	26			1 2			X	0																0	
6 Saturday	27											1 2													X

Figure 8.1 Fourteen-day sleep diary: treatment with modafinil and fluoxetine. Blue, awake; pink, asleep; X, cataplexia episode; O, sleep attack; 1, modafinil; 2, fluoxetine.

Sodium oxybate has become available only relatively recently and represents a significant advance in the treatment of narcolepsy with cataplexy, as it is highly effective for the treatment of the latter. Sodium oxybate is the only FDA-approved drug for the treatment of cataplexy. It is a $GABA_B$ receptor agonist, although the exact mechanism of anticataplectic activity remains unknown. Abrupt cessation of oxybate administration leads to a recurrence of cataplexy without rebound phenomenon and no reported tolerance.

The transition from antidepressants to sodium oxybate was made after a gradual withdrawal of the antidepressant and a washout, as was reported in the clinical trial. Sometimes the treatment of cataplexy with sodium oxybate can be initiated while the patient remains on antidepressants. Once the optimal dose of sodium oxybate has been achieved, the tapering or withdrawal of antidepressants may be desirable. Further studies are needed to examine possible interactions and side effects of co-administration of antidepressants and sodium oxybate.

Antidepressant compounds have been used for the treatment of cataplexy before sodium oxybate became available, as was apparent in this case. Tricyclic antidepressants were the first drugs discovered to have anticataplectic activity and have been used for 40 years. Later, other types of antidepressants were tested as they became available. Selective serotonin reuptake inhibitors (SSRIs) were introduced in the treatment of cataplexy, as well as inhibitors of monoamine oxidase A (selegiline, mazindol), venlafaxine, viloxazine, reboxetine and atomoxetine. Antidepressants block the reuptake of norepinephrine and serotonin neurotransmitters, increasing muscle tone and suppressing REM activity. This patient took clomipramine, the most effective tricyclic antidepressant REM-sleep suppressor. It gave rise to tolerance after 16 months of administration, a well-known occurrence. Fluoxetine and all SSRIs in general are less efficacious than tricyclic antidepressants, as became apparent in this case.

Pearls and gold

Circadian dysrhythmia is an aggravating factor in narcolepsy.

Sodium oxybate successfully reduces cataplexy and improves other symptoms of narcolepsy such as excessive sleepiness, hypnagogic hallucinations and sleep paralysis, even in the presence of an aggravating risk factor such as circadian dysrhythmia.

A tailored titration of sodium oxybate administration is feasible when aggravating factors intervene. The short half-life of sodium oxybate facilitates this process.

SUGGESTED READING

REVIEW

Wise MS, Arand Dl, Auger RR, Brooks SN, Watson NF. Treatment of narcolepsy and other hypersomnias of central origin. An American Academy of Sleep Medicine Review. *Sleep* 2007; **30**: 1712–27.

GENERAL

AASM (American Academy of Sleep Medicine). *International Classification of Sleep Disorders*, revised: *Diagnostic and Coding Manual.* Westchester, Illinois: American Academy of Sleep Medicine, 2001.

AASM (American Academy of Sleep Medicine). *International Classification of Sleep Disorders*, 2nd edn.: *Diagnostic and Coding Manual.* Westchester, Illinois: American Academy of Sleep Medicine, 2005.

Anic-Labat S, Guilleminault C, Kraemer HC, *et al.* Validation of a cataplexy questionnaire in 983 sleep-disorders patients. *Sleep* 1999; **22**: 77–87.

Hayduk RM, Erman M, Mitler MM. Treatment of cataplexy with sodium oxybate: transition from tricyclic antidepressants (TCAs) and selective serotonin reuptake inhibitors (SSRIs). *Sleep* **2** (abstract supplement), 2003.

Hublin C, Kaprio J, Partinen M, Koskenvuo M, Heikkila K. The Ullanlinna Narcolepsy Scale: validation of a measure of symptoms in the narcoleptic syndrome. *J Sleep Res* 1994; **3**: 52–9.

Parkes JD, Chen SY, Clift SJ, Dahlitz MJ, Dunn G. The clinical diagnosis of the narcoleptic syndrome. *J Sleep Res* 1998; **7**: 41–52.

Thorpy M. Therapeutic advances in narcolepsy. *Sleep Med* 2007; **8**: 427–40.

Vignatelli L, D'Alessandro R, Candelise L. Antidepresant drugs for narcolepsy. *Cochrane Database of Systematic Reviews* 2008, Issue 1. Art. No CD003724. DOI: 10.1002/14651858. CD003724. pub3.

Part IV

Parasomnias

A. REM-sleep-associated parasomnias

Case 9

Extreme dreams
Philip King

Clinical history

A 55-year-old woman reported that for the previous 6 years she had been having episodes at night where she had dreams that often had a fearful content. According to her husband, some of these were associated with her kicking, punching, shouting and making noises. She had had three episodes where she had injured herself and, following these, she recounted the dreams to her husband and they reported on what happened. In one, she was pursued by crocodiles and had launched herself out of the bed into an en suite bathroom about 2 m away. She sustained significant bruising. In another, she dreamed a man was coming to "get her" and she later found she had broken several of her toenails and injured her toes kicking the bedside table with what appeared to be defensive movements. The third episode with injury was 6 weeks prior to assessment, when she was on a cruise ship in Greece. She woke and found herself on the floor of a cupboard at the end of the bunk. She had what she described as a "carpet burn" on her face and the left side of the body and she had injured her back and hip. She reported a fearful dream but did not recollect the details at the interview. All the episodes occurred after she had been asleep for at least 2 hours.

She and her husband reported dreaming, talking, shouting, punching or kicking movements increasing in frequency over 6 years such that they were now occurring about every second night. The content was varied, but when they discussed the episodes, the vocalization and motor activity seemed appropriate to the dream. Occasionally, she would have two episodes in one night.

She snored occasionally, but did not wake up short of breath, choking or with a feeling she had been snoring, and her husband had not witnessed apneas. She was not sleepy during the day.

She had had a restless feeling in her legs for the previous 6 years. She described a crawling feeling inside her skin. She wriggled her feet every 30 seconds or so in

Case Studies in Sleep Neurology: Common and Uncommon Presentations, ed. A. Culebras. Published by Cambridge University Press. © Cambridge University Press 2010.

order to relieve the symptoms when they occurred. The episodes were worst lying in bed prior to sleep, but also occurred when watching television, at the movies or on plane trips. Her symptoms were worse when she was anemic prior to bowel cancer being diagnosed 9 months prior to the initial assessment, and they settled back to baseline over several months following a right hemicolectomy for resection of the tumor.

About 3 years prior to the initial assessment, she first noted her voice had become "croaky." A year later she first noted waking occasionally with excessive saliva around her mouth. Between 1 and 2 years prior to her presentation, she first noted an intermittent tremor affecting the left foot. She subsequently noticed a tremor affecting the left hand. Both had got worse over the 6 months prior to the initial assessment. She had also noticed when typing that her left little finger "wandered around" and she noted difficulty striking the correct key. She thought she was clumsier than usual. She had not noted any changes to her walking, running or ability to roll over in bed or to perform fine movements such as doing up buttons or putting on makeup. She had noted pain and subsequent numbness around the heel of the left foot 2 years before the initial assessment and the numbness had persisted.

Her only medication was estrogen hormone replacement; she had stopped smoking 6 years previously and her alcohol consumption was about three standard drinks on 2 days per week. The episodes at night were not related to whether or not she drank alcohol. The patient and her son had had episodes of sleepwalking when they were young, but there was no other family history of parasomnia. Three of her sisters had had breast cancer.

Examination

On examination she was anxious and cried during the interview. There was an intermittent tremor of the left hand and foot at rest. It was slightly worse doing mental arithmetic. The tremor was not apparent with the upper limbs stretched out in front of her or with finger–nose testing and other movements. There was mild bradykinesia of the left fingers and rigidity in the left upper limb. She did not swing the left upper limb as well as the right when she walked, but her gait was otherwise normal. The reflexes were all present and symmetrical, and the responses on plantar stimulation were flexor. There was reduced touch sensation around the left heel, but sensory examination was otherwise normal. Her voice was slightly hoarse but of normal volume. Eye movements and other cranial nerve examinations were normal. There was no drop in blood pressure from the lying to the sitting position.

Special studies

An MRI scan of the brain, EEG and overnight polysomnography (PSG) were performed.

Results of studies

The brain MRI showed some non-specific white matter changes that were thought most likely to be age related. The EEG showed several runs of temporal slowing during drowsiness, shifting sides. No definite focal abnormalities or epileptiform activity were seen.

Overnight video-PSG showed increased tonic and phasic EMG activity in the submental EMG recording and increased phasic EMG activity in the tibialis anterior EMG (Figure 9.1). Frequent arousals and brief awakenings were noted from REM sleep. Talking and some upper limb movements were noted for a few seconds on several occasions during REM sleep, but no shouting or other loud vocalization, kicking, punching or violent activity was noted. Periodic limb movements of sleep (PLMS) were identified (38 per hour), but there was no significant apnea (the respiratory disturbance index was zero) and no significant O_2 desaturation.

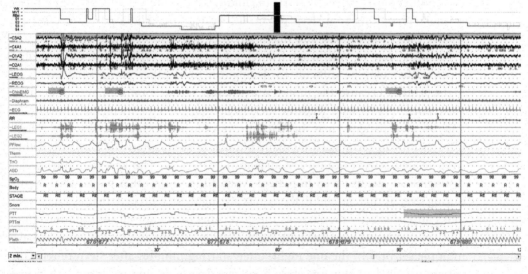

Figure 9.1   REM sleep in the patient with 2 minutes of recording displayed. The hypnogram on the top shows sleep stage. Note the prominent submental EMG activity with phasic and tonic features and the prominent phasic EMG activity in the tibialis anterior muscle recording channels (LEG1 and LEG2). LEOG/REOG, left/right electro-oculogram; RR, respiratory rate; THO, thorax; ABD, abdomen; SpO$_2$, arterial oxyhemoglobin saturation.

Question

How many sleep-related disorders does this patient have?

Diagnosis

The examiner felt that the night episodes were REM-sleep behavior disorder (RBD) and that the patient had early Parkinson's disease and restless legs syndrome (RLS).

The differential diagnosis of paroxysmal nocturnal events includes parasomnia, seizures during sleep or a psychogenic disturbance. Parasomnia classification is usually based on the sleep phase during which the parasomnia occurs. NREM parasomnias include disorders of arousal (confusional arousals, sleep terrors and sleepwalking). There is a genetic predisposition to these, and members of the same family may exhibit different combinations of the named disorders. The content of NREM parasomnia events is typically variable, as it is in RBD. Unlike RBD, dream recall is usually absent or very vague, often involving shadowy figures in the bedroom, but the content of both is typically fearful. A common error is to assume that any dream recall excludes NREM parasomnia because dreaming is usually associated with REM sleep, but this is not the case. NREM parasomnia most frequently starts in childhood, but there is a bias to adult onset in those presenting to a sleep physician because the childhood-onset cases are usually easier to diagnose and the differential diagnosis in adults is broader.

Seizures seen in nocturnal frontal lobe epilepsy (NFLE) are sleep-related seizures that may be difficult to distinguish from other paroxysmal events at night. This is because the motor activity and vocalization may resemble other paroxysmal events with features such as cycling movements of the lower limbs and because patients may be partially responsive during the seizures. These features are not recognized by many physicians as suggestive of a seizure. Other sleep-related seizures cause less diagnostic difficulty. The key component that distinguishes seizures seen in patients with NFLE from other paroxysmal events during sleep is that, in NFLE, the events are highly stereotyped, that is, each event looks almost exactly the same as the next. This is true for all seizures, including those particularly associated with sleep. Usually but not always, patients will have multiple seizures in the one night, often starting minutes after sleep onset. Our patient usually had only one episode every 2 days or so, and never more than two episodes per night, while the behavior and vocalization during the events were not stereotyped. Nocturnal frontal lobe epilepsy may be familial. If stereotypy of the events is not appreciated, there may be confusion with NREM parasomnia, which may also be familial, as noted above. REM-sleep behavior disorder is not usually familial.

An event from a psychogenic disturbance was felt unlikely, but must always be considered in the differential diagnosis of paroxysmal nocturnal events. It is generally believed that patients with these disturbances rouse and the behavior occurs during the wake or drowsy state and not that the psychogenic state causes arousal from otherwise normal sleep. Return of alpha and other signs of arousal are usually seen prior to an event, and where the EEG is not obscured by muscle and movement artifacts it will show wakeful or drowsy patterns throughout the episode. This could cause diagnostic difficulty with RBD because alpha-like activity is expected in REM sleep. A sudden brief return of the submental EMG to that seen in normal REM sleep may be seen during RBD episodes and, if present, would suggest that the patient is actually in REM sleep. RBD is only seen in REM sleep, whereas events from a psychogenic disturbance may occur following an arousal from REM or NREM sleep. Frank wakefulness prior to an event in the appropriate setting strongly suggests a psychogenic cause.

General remarks

REM-sleep behavior disorder was recognized as a distinct clinical entity only relatively recently by Schenck, Mahowald and co-workers. Patients literally act out their dreams. The dreams characteristically have a violent content. The vocalization usually consists of shouting and swearing, even in those not accustomed to swearing during wakefulness. The motor activity is usually violent and consists of punching and kicking. Patients may be roused much more easily during and after these events than patients with NREM parasomnia, and in the morning they are able to report a dream corresponding to the vocalization and motor activity. The dreams are usually variable in content and recall is much more elaborate than that seen in NREM parasomnia. Bed partners are often injured, more frequently as an innocent "bystander" than by being incorporated into the dream, although the latter may occur. The activity usually takes place in the bed, but patients may fall or launch themselves out of the bed. These more dramatic episodes are more likely to be brought to the attention of the sleep physician because they are memorable and more likely to lead to injury. Ambulation is very rare and if it occurs it is only for a step or two. Beyond this, the diagnosis is much more likely to be sleepwalking or a seizure.

The history from the patient and bed partner is crucial for the correct diagnosis of nocturnal events. A home video of the events is always very helpful. It may be regarded as an extension of the history: "a picture tells a thousand words." The video should be examined for stereotypy and also for dystonic movements or other features that may suggest a seizure. A careful neurological examination should always be performed. In this case, the neurological examination was very helpful, but often it is entirely normal. The role of imaging studies such as an MRI scan of the brain depends on availability and certainty of diagnosis. An MRI scan showing a frontal lesion, mesial temporal sclerosis or other temporal lesion would make one more alert for a seizure diagnosis. Pontine atrophy may be seen in multiple system atrophy (see below), but this is not an early feature. It is often difficult to obtain an EEG of optimum quality to look for interictal abnormalities during the night sleep study because of noise and artifacts from additional recording equipment and the environment of the sleep laboratory. If so, it is usually helpful to perform a daytime sleep-deprived sleep EEG in a neurological setting in order to look for interictal abnormalities (spikes, sharp waves, focal slowing) that may indicate a higher-than-normal chance of seizures at other times. The purpose of the sleep deprivation is to make sleep more likely during the day and to increase the likelihood of seeing spikes or sharp waves, whether or not the patient sleeps, not an expectation that the patient will have an event during the EEG.

Nocturnal video-PSG is now considered an essential part of making a diagnosis of RBD. In addition to the possibility of recording an event, a reduction of the usual atonia seen in the submental EMG and an increase in phasic submental and/or limb EMG compared with that seen in normal REM sleep is usually seen. These findings are observed whether or not the patient has a RBD episode. Such findings in REM sleep do not prove but are a point in favor of a diagnosis of RBD. If an event or events with violent motor activity and vocalization is recorded in REM sleep, RBD is very likely. In the patient's sleep study, no typical major episodes were seen in REM sleep, but vocalization and some motor movements were noted. This or no abnormal motor activity at all is common, particularly when the frequency of major events obtained from the patient's history is low. In this situation, the REM-sleep abnormalities as seen in the polysomnogram are very helpful. REM-sleep behavior disorder only occurs during REM sleep, but occasionally patients who have features of REM and NREM parasomnias may be seen. Very few epileptic seizures occur exclusively in REM sleep.

The largest series of patients with RBD who have had neuropathological studies performed has been updated recently and now includes 36 patients. All but one has shown evidence of synuclein inclusions in neurons. The patient without synuclein inclusions had progressive supranuclear palsy, a tauopathy. The synucleinopathies (diseases characterized by synuclein inclusions) are Parkinson's disease, multiple system atrophy and dementia with Lewy bodies. Synuclein is part of the Lewy body seen in these patients. It is now recognized that RBD may occur up to 10 years or so before symptoms of one of the synucleinopathies becomes evident, and occasionally the time interval may be longer. Thus, many cases of RBD previously assumed to be idiopathic are not so on follow-up. The patient had symptoms suggestive of Parkinson's disease, and in her case a diagnosis of RBD and Parkinson's disease was made at the same time, an uncommon situation. Close follow-up of all patients with apparent "idiopathic" RBD is mandatory to monitor for the development of Parkinson's disease, multiple system atrophy or dementia with Lewy bodies. Unfortunately, at present, there is no treatment that prevents progression of these disorders. If such a treatment is developed, an exciting possibility will be a trial to treat patients with RBD before the clinical manifestations of a synucleinopathy develop.

The patient responded well to clonazepam at bedtime, which is the usual treatment. Other shorter-acting benzodiazepines may be used if daytime sedation occurs with clonazepam. A good starting dose is 0.25–0.5 mg. This can be increased by 0.25–0.5 mg increments every week or so if necessary and if tolerated, and depending on the frequency of events. "Go low, go slow" is the best approach. This ensures that the lowest effective dose is used and minimizes the risk of the patient refusing to continue the drug because of excessive daytime sedation, a "drugged" feeling or other side effects. Doses higher than 2 mg are usually unnecessary and often are not tolerated. Clonazepam makes sleep apnea worse and this must be watched for, particularly if higher doses of clonazepam are used. Melatonin 3–12 mg at night may be used if clonazepam is unsuccessful or not tolerated. Levodopa or pramipexole may be effective in some patients. Tricyclic antidepressants, mirtazapine and selective serotonin and noradrenaline reuptake inhibitors, especially venlafaxine, may cause or exacerbate RBD and they should be withdrawn if possible prior to considering additional medication. Withdrawal of the medications used to treat RBD listed above may also trigger RBD.

The patient was not bothered greatly by her parkinsonian symptoms and, following a discussion, it was decided not to initiate drug treatment immediately. A "croaky voice" is an uncommon feature of Parkinson's disease and it raises the possibility of multiple system atrophy where voice changes and respiratory stridor are commonly seen due to paresis of the vocal cord abductor muscles. The other features and time course were, however, more in keeping with Parkinson's disease. The left heel numbness may represent a focal onset of symptoms of a peripheral neuropathy. Restless legs syndrome (RLS) and PLMS may occur secondary to a peripheral neuropathy. In this case, the patient's restless legs symptoms were not severe enough to warrant drug treatment. Nerve conduction studies, serum ferritin and other tests are planned in order to investigate this further.

Pearls and gold

Patients with RBD may be roused much more easily during and after events than patients with NREM parasomnia, and in the morning they are able to report a dream corresponding to the vocalization and motor activity.

Ambulation is very rare in RBD and, if it occurs, it is only for a step or two.

The largest series of patients with RBD who have had neuropathological studies performed comprises 36 patients. All but one has shown evidence of synuclein inclusions in neurons.

Close follow-up of all patients with apparent idiopathic RBD is mandatory to monitor for the development of Parkinson's disease, multiple system atrophy or dementia with Lewy bodies.

SUGGESTED READING

HISTORICAL

Schenck CH, Bundlie SR, Ettinger MG, Mahowald MW. Chronic behavioral disorders of human REM sleep: a new category of parasomnia. *Sleep* 1986; **9**: 293–308.

GENERAL

Boeve BF, Silber MH, Saper CB, *et al.* Pathophysiology of REM sleep behaviour disorder and relevance to neurodegenerative disease. *Brain* 2007; **130**: 2770–88.

Iranzo A, Santamaría J, Tolosa E. The clinical and pathophysiological relevance of REM sleep behavior disorder in neurodegenerative diseases. *Sleep Med Rev* 2009; **13**: 385–401.

Schenck CH, Bundlie SR, Mahowald MW. Delayed emergence of a parkinsonian disorder in 38% of 29 older men initially diagnosed with idiopathic rapid eye movement sleep behavior disorder. *Neurology* 1996; **46**: 388–93.

Odd sleep-related behaviors

Hrayr P. Attarian .

Clinical history

Mr. C. was a 27-year-old man who presented to the sleep clinic with odd behaviors during sleep for the past year. The current problem started about a year prior to his visit, when he moved in with his girlfriend of 2 years. He had two types of events. The first occurred later on during the night and was associated with anxiety-producing and scary dreams. He tended to be very active during these, often grabbing his girlfriend and shaking her and trying to punch her or kicking the dog, but rarely leaving the bed. When aroused, he clearly recalled dreams of being engaged in a fist fight with someone or being on the football field trying to kick the ball. These events occurred about once a month and had remained stable in frequency throughout the past year. The other type occurred earlier on during the night and was associated with yelling and screaming and often ended out of bed. On occasions, he sat up in bed, screamed his nephew's name and got out of bed looking for him; during another, he tried to throw a television set across the room. It took quite a bit of effort to awaken him from these events and he had no recollection of the spells or his dreams. Initially, after his move, the episodes occurred every day; however, gradually they abated to once a week at the most.

Mr. C. was a known sleeptalker and sleepwalker since mid- to late childhood. In his adult years, the sleepwalking condition decreased in frequency to one or two events per year. During sleepwalking, he never left the house, but he frequently woke up on the couch or somewhere other than his bed. He was very difficult to arouse during sleepwalking and had no recollection the next day of having done it, and was frequently confused to find himself elsewhere in the house.

At the time of presentation, the patient had a consistent bedtime of 11.30 pm. He usually watched television for 15–30 minutes before falling asleep. He slept right through until 7.30–8 am, awakening spontaneously but feeling a bit groggy in the mornings. He did not have daytime sleepiness. The Epworth Sleepiness

Case Studies in Sleep Neurology: Common and Uncommon Presentations, ed. A. Culebras. Published by Cambridge University Press. © Cambridge University Press 2010.

Scale score was 4/24 (normal; see Appendix) and he did not have fatigue. He was an intermittent snorer, but denied observed pauses in breathing, and denied awakenings with heartburn, headache or dry mouth. He denied night sweats, leg jerks, hypnagogic hallucinations, sleep paralysis, tongue biting, bowel/bladder incontinence or generalized tonic/clonic movement during the night. He also denied a history of febrile seizures, perinatal injury, meningitis, concussion or head trauma. He denied drinking alcohol, using tobacco or illicit drugs. He drank one can of highly caffeinated soda a day in the morning, but more out of habit and because he liked the taste than from the need to be awake.

Examination

The patient was a healthy-looking male sitting in the chair in no apparent distress. He weighed 95.5 kg and measured 175 cm. His BMI was 30.1 kg/m^2. His general examination was otherwise normal. A neurological examination was likewise normal.

Special studies

Nocturnal polysomnography (PSG) with additional all-night 16-channel EEG running concomitantly with the PSG was obtained (Figures 10.1 and 10.2).

Question

What is your diagnosis: sleepwalking or REM-sleep behavior disorder (RBD)?

Results of studies

The patient slept for 406 minutes out of 432 minutes in bed, resulting in a normal sleep efficiency of 94%. Sleep-onset latency and REM-sleep latency were both normal at 8 and 79 minutes, respectively. Sleep-stage distribution was normal with 28% REM sleep, 4% stage N1, 62% stage N2 and 6% stage N3. Sleep was minimally fragmented with an arousal index just about normal at eight arousals per hour, which appeared to be spontaneous in nature. There was no evidence of obstructive sleep apnea (OSA) with normal breathing and normal O$_2$ saturation during sleep averaging 93% with a nadir of 90% and a desaturation index of zero. Average heart rate was 55 bpm. There were no periodic limb movements. He had increased EMG activity during REM sleep associated with talking and brief movements of his arms and legs. He also had sleeptalking and some movement arising out of stage N2 sleep. No EEG abnormalities were present.

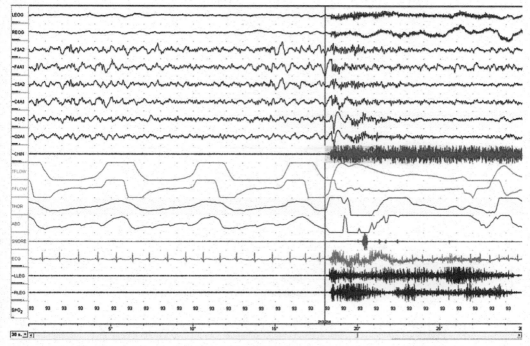

Figure 10.1 Event from NREM sleep. The patient is in stage N2 sleep and starting at the 21st second he is attempting to get out of bed while still in NREM sleep. Note the sudden increase in muscle tone in the chin and right and left leg EMG channels. LEOG/REOG, left/right electro-oculogram; TFLOW, thermistor, flow monitor; PFLOW, pressure flow monitor; THO, thorax; ABD, abdomen; SpO$_2$, arterial oxyhemoglobin saturation.

Diagnosis

Given these results, a diagnosis of parasomnia overlap disorder was made. ICSD-2 (AASM, 2005) includes the overlap disorder under "Parasomnias usually associated with REM sleep."

Follow-up

At the follow-up visit, the specialist gave Mr. C. and his girlfriend an overview of the test results, a prognosis of the disorder and suggestions for management. He explained that people with parasomnia overlap disorder have clinical features of RBD, as well as a disorder of arousal. Mr. C. had a history of somnambulism, as well as dream-enacting behavior, and on PSG two events were captured, one out of NREM sleep and one with increased tone out of REM sleep. The specialist prescribed clonazepam 0.5 mg at bedtime. Mr. C. was instructed that clonazepam may cause morning grogginess and that there is a low incidence of tolerance and

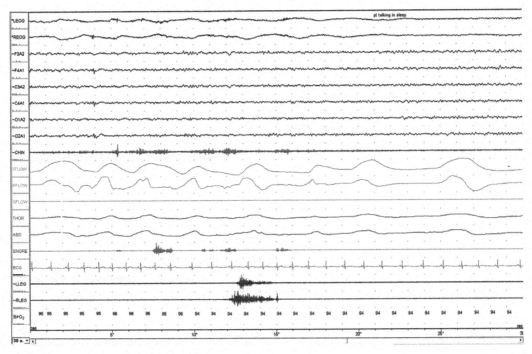

Figure 10.2 Event from REM sleep. The patient is in REM sleep. Note the preserved muscle tone. He is talking and gesturing. See Figure 10.1 legend for abbreviations.

addiction with clonazepam. Mr. C. was also informed of the possibility of developing Parkinsonism in the future and that Parkinsonism is observed in one-third of males over the age of 50, on average 13 years after the diagnosis of RBD. He was also informed that, as his condition is a variant of RBD, the association is not as well defined. Serial neurological examinations were recommended annually during follow-up visits to identify Parkinsonism early. His history and a thorough neurological examination ruled out the other associated conditions listed below.

General remarks

The ICSD-2 (AASM, 2005) defines parasomnia overlap disorder as consisting of both RBD and a disorder of arousal (sleepwalking, confusional arousal or sleep terror). The diagnosis is made when diagnostic criteria of both conditions have been met. Parasomnia overlap disorder, like RBD, has a male predominance but a lesser one. It has an earlier age of onset, with most cases occurring in adolescence, but it has been known to occur in any age group. Associated conditions include narcolepsy, multiple sclerosis, head trauma, brain tumor, Machado–Joseph disease, nocturnal paroxysmal atrial fibrillation, Möbius syndrome and various psychiatric conditions and their pharmacotherapies.

The first report of the co-existence of both conditions was by Bokey (1993) from Australia. He described a case of both conditions co-existing in a 49-year-old Vietnam War veteran who was previously diagnosed with conversion disorder for these sleep-related unusual behaviors. After undergoing PSG, both types of events were captured and he was treated with clonazepam with resolution of the events.

Schenck *et al.* (1997) coined the term parasomnia overlap disorder in their 1997 paper where they described 33 cases, all confirmed by PSG to have both conditions, over a period of 8 years. The mean age was 33.8±13.9 years with a range of 5–72 years. The mean age of onset, however, was 14.6±16.3 years with a range of 1–66 years. Twenty-three (69.7%) were male and ten (30.3%) were female. Two-thirds (22 subjects) had an idiopathic form and one-third (11 subjects) had a symptomatic form. Six were significantly associated with one of the neurological conditions mentioned above, one with atrial fibrillation, two with psychiatric problems, and two had both a psychiatric condition and head trauma. Ninety percent of the treated subjects had complete control of symptoms lasting from 6 months up to 9 years. The treatments used were clonazepam, alprazolam and carbamazepine, and, in the case of a 5-year-old, image-guided self-hypnosis. In 2004, two other cases of parasomnia overlap disorder were reported in patients with Harlequin syndrome (Horner's syndrome, hypohydrosis and contralateral facial flushing).

The proposed pathophysiology is thought to be motor dyscontrol during both REM and NREM sleep. In most cases, the anatomical location of this dysfunction appears to be the brainstem and particularly the midbrain; however, the pons and medulla play a major role in generating both REM sleep atonia and phasic motor activation during REM sleep. The association between parasomnia overlap disorder and autonomic disorders such as Harlequin syndrome further suggests this. In most cases, the anatomical location of this dysfunction appears to be the brainstem. This would also explain the higher prevalence of RBD in Parkinson's disease patients and the occurrence of parasomnia overlap disorder in patients with brainstem disorders, including multiple sclerosis, Möbius syndrome and traumatic brain injury involving the brainstem. In 2007, an increased prevalence of sleepwalking was also reported with Parkinson's disease. Parkinson's disease-associated neurodegenerative changes at the brainstem level can affect the "ascending" control of state transition leading to dissociated arousals from NREM sleep as well as REM sleep. Rarely, the co-existence of both conditions could be due to psychiatric disorders that increase the risk of NREM parasomnias and their treatment with selective serotonin reuptake inhibitors (SSRIs) or selective norepinephrine reuptake inhibitors (SNRIs) that can cause RBD.

There is also a familial and genetic component to parasomnia overlap disorder. Schenck *et al.* (1997) identified a family where three adult first-degree relations were documented to have RBD, sleepwalking, sleep terrors, narcolepsy and periodic/aperiodic limb movements of NREM sleep in various combinations.

DNA samples from patients with sleepwalking and controls were collected from four sleep centers in Europe. The analysis showed a significant increase in the DQB1*0501 and DQB1*0402 allele frequency in sleepwalkers. DQB1*05 is also associated with RBD, so there is evidence that REM sleep-associated parasomnias such as RBD and NREM parasomnias such as sleepwalking may share a genetic background, as exemplified by individuals affected by parasomnia overlap disorder.

As in other parasomnias, the differential diagnosis includes nocturnal seizures, medication effects and any of the other parasomnia subtypes. A full-head EEG and PSG are often helpful to capture events during the night of the study. Alternatively, if there is preservation of muscle tone in REM sleep and the patient has a history of events suggestive of partial arousal disorder, then the diagnosis can be made with greater certainty.

Treatment includes benzodiazepines, primarily clonazepam, and behavioral therapy methods such as self-hypnosis, often in combination. Other treatments that have been reported to be helpful have been alprazolam, low-dose tricyclic antidepressants and carbamazepine.

Prognosis is unknown, but careful follow-up is recommended to help with early detection of Parkinsonian disorder or other degenerative neurological disorders that are known to be associated with RBD.

In conclusion, parasomnia overlap disorder is a variant of RBD; it appears to affect a younger age group with male predilection. A variety of psychiatric, medical and neurological conditions can be associated with it. The treatment is similar to that of RBD.

Pearls and gold

Parasomnia overlap disorder consists of both RBD and a disorder of arousal – sleepwalking, confusional arousal or sleep terror.

One-third of patients may have an associated serious neurological condition.

In most cases, the anatomical location of the dysfunction appears to be the brainstem.

Parasomnia overlap disorder responds to the administration of clonazepam.

SUGGESTED READING

HISTORICAL

Bokey K. Conversion disorder revisited: severe parasomnia discovered. *Aust N Z J Psychiatry* 1993; **27**: 694.

REVIEW

Schenck CH, Mahowald MW. Rapid eye movement sleep parasomnias. *Neurol Clin* 2005; **23**: 1107–26.

GENERAL

AASM (American Academy of Sleep Medicine). *International Classification of Sleep Disorders,* 2nd edn.: *Diagnostic and Coding Manual.* Westchester, Illinois: American Academy of Sleep Medicine, 2005.

Kushida CA, Clerk AA, Kirsch CM, *et al.* Prolonged confusion with nocturnal wandering arising from NREM and REM sleep: a case report. *Sleep* 1995; **18**: 757–64.

Lombardi C, Vetrugni R, Provini F, *et al.* Harlequin syndrome: an association with overlap parasomnia. *J Neurol Neurosurg Psychiatry* 2004; **75**: 341–2.

Mahowald MW, Schenck CH. Dissociated states of wakefulness and sleep. *Neurology* 1992; **42**: 44–52.

Schenck CH, Boyd JL, Mahowald MW. A parasomnia overlap disorder involving sleepwalking, sleep terrors, and REM sleep behavior disorder in 33 polysomnographically confirmed cases. *Sleep* 1997; **20**: 972–81.

Young P. Genetic aspects of parasomnias. *Somnologie* 2008; **12**: 7–13.

Paralyzed and unable to breathe

Hrayr P. Attarian

Clinical history

Mr. N. was a 56-year-old man who presented to the sleep clinic complaining of frequent episodes of feeling paralyzed as he was going to sleep. He would wake up with palpitations, shortness of breath and the feeling that someone or something was sitting on his chest. He was unable to move, scream, open his eyes or take a deep breath during these episodes, despite his best efforts. He described the overall feeling as being "dead." This was associated with severe fear, even though at the back of his mind he knew he was going to come out of it "all right." He had been having these events on and off since his early 20s. Initially, they used to occur sporadically when short of sleep or if he was affected by physical or psychosocial stressors. Around the age of 48, they started occurring more frequently, and at the time of his presentation they had been occurring 4–6 times a week. Two years before, he had gone to his primary care physician voicing this complaint in addition to non-restorative sleep and loud snoring. Polysomnography (PSG) done at the time had shown mild obstructive sleep apnea syndrome (OSAS) with an apnea–hypopnea index (AHI) of 11 per hour (Figure 11.1). After failing a brief trial of continuous positive airway pressure (CPAP), he had undergone an uvulopalatopharyngoplasty surgical intervention. Repeat PSG 3 months after the intervention showed resolution of the OSAS with an AHI of 3 per hour. His fatigue also improved, but he continued to snore and, most importantly, he continued to experience the frequent episodes of paralysis.

He usually went to bed at about 11.30 pm and fell asleep right away, unless he experienced an episode of paralysis. After an episode, he had such severe palpitations and agitation that it took him about 30 minutes to calm down and fall asleep again. He woke up at 7 am on weekdays and 9 am on weekends. Sleep was interrupted by two bathroom visits, after which he was able to fall back to sleep with relative ease. He only experienced these episodes at sleep onset, never in the middle of the night or in the morning, and never during naps, which he rarely took.

Case Studies in Sleep Neurology: Common and Uncommon Presentations, ed. A. Culebras. Published by Cambridge University Press. © Cambridge University Press 2010.

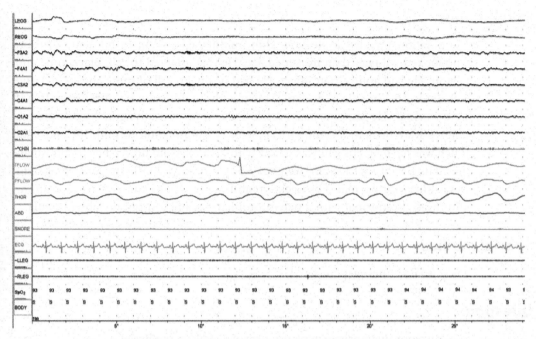

Figure 11.1 The epoch before the patient woke up stating he had just had an episode of sleep paralysis. Note the faster frequencies more characteristic of wakefulness, mixed with REM sleep-like activity together with atonia. LEOG/REOG, left/right electro-oculogram; TFLOW, thermistor flow monitor; PFLOW, pressure flow monitor; THOR, thorax; ABD, abdomen; SpO₂, arterial oxyhemoglobin saturation.

He denied otherwise having trouble falling asleep or staying asleep. He denied excessive daytime sleepiness (EDS); his Epworth Sleepiness Scale score was 5 (see Appendix). He denied enuresis, cataplexy and hypnagogic hallucinations, either independent or associated with the periods of paralysis. He could no longer identify any triggers for these episodes. He did not have any lifestyle or dietary habits that made these more frequent. No other complaints were reported by him.

His past medical history was not significant. He was not allergic to any medications and was not taking any. He was a physician's assistant in a primary care clinic and was married with two adult children. He did not use tobacco, drank alcohol rarely and had two cups of coffee a day. He did not abuse illicit drugs. He had heard his father complain occasionally of similar episodes of paralysis in the past and his daughter had also mentioned similar episodes to him.

Examination

Examination revealed a pleasant, thin, middle-aged man, in no acute distress, who looked younger than his stated age. He was oriented to self, place, time and person. He had appropriate affect. He had normal recall of three objects at 1 and 5 minutes. He was able to do serial sevens without difficulty. Cranial nerves II–XII were normal. He had normal muscle bulk, tone and strength. Muscle stretch reflexes were brisk and symmetrical. Sensory examination to pinprick and light touch was normal. His gait was steady with no ataxia and no cerebellar abnormalities. His height was 178 cm, weight 75.5 kg and BMI 23.8 kg/m^2. His vital signs were otherwise normal. His neck circumference was 41 cm. A general examination was also normal with a patent oropharynx and a surgically absent uvula.

Special studies

No special studies were ordered.

Question

What is your diagnosis: narcolepsy or isolated sleep paralysis?

Diagnosis

Based on the history, the diagnosis of isolated or familial sleep paralysis was made and the patient was started on clomipramine 25 mg at bedtime.

Follow-up

The patient came back after 6 weeks of taking clomipramine 25 mg at bedtime and stated that the episodes had indeed decreased in frequency to once or twice a week but that he wanted better control of the events. The dose was increased to 50 mg at bedtime and at the 1-year follow-up visit, he reported that his episodes were completely controlled and in fact he had had only one since increasing the dose to 50 mg. He had no adverse effects from the medication.

General remarks

Sleep paralysis has been part of the folklore of many cultures (from North America to Asia and Africa) under different names and has often been attributed to paranormal activity. The first description of it in the medical literature, as "night palsy," was in 1876 (Mitchell, 1876). Sleep paralysis is a recognized clinical entity that falls under the category of REM sleep parasomnias. ICSD-2 (AASM, 2005), defines recurrent isolated sleep paralysis as an inability to perform voluntary movements occurring at sleep onset or when awakening in the absence of a diagnosis of narcolepsy.

Isolated paralysis occurs most often when awakening; this is the postdormital or hypnopompic type. The familial and sleep paralysis associated with narcolepsy tend to occur more frequently while falling asleep; this is the predormital or hypnagogic type. Both hypnopompic and hypnagogic types, however, can occur in all three syndromes: isolated and familial sleep paralysis and that associated with narcolepsy. The person is unable to move their limbs or facial muscles or to vocalize. Although there is a subjective sense of shortness of breath, respiratory muscles are spared. The person experiencing it is always fully awake and can easily recall the event afterwards. The episode lasts seconds to minutes (average duration 4 minutes) and usually resolves spontaneously but may be aborted by sensory, usually tactile, stimulation. Intense anxiety is often a feature of the event and hallucinations can accompany sleep paralysis up to three-quarters of the time. Relapses can occur, especially if lying in the supine position. The frequency of the episodes is also higher in supine sleepers and those who experience it at the beginning and middle of the night rather than the end of the night. Timing also affects the severity of the anxiety, with sleep-onset episodes being more anxiety provoking.

Rare isolated sleep paralysis, often occurring only once or twice in a lifetime, has been reported in up to 40% of people. Males and females are affected equally and the peak incidence is in the late teens. Recurrent isolated sleep paralysis has a prevalence of 5%. Twenty percent of cases are familial. Patients who experience recurrent sleep paralysis have a mean prevalence of 6.7 episodes in a lifetime, 2.02 per year and 0.5 per month. According to Ohaeri et al. (2004), 2.7% of these patients have sleep paralysis at least once per week, 18.2% once per month and 75.5% less than once per month. Sleep paralysis associated with narcolepsy tends to occur nightly at certain periods and to become rare at others. Some narcolepsy patients tend to sleep upright to avoid the frequent episodes of sleep paralysis.

In addition to narcolepsy, familial sleep paralysis (with a possible maternal transmission) can be associated with sleep deprivation. Other causes of sleep paralysis include schizophrenia, Wilson's disease and bipolar affective disorder.

Sleep paralysis is a condition characterized by a pathological dissociation between level of alertness and the generalized muscle atonia typical of REM sleep. When captured in PSG, athough this is rare, it shows a dissociated state of mixed wake and REM-sleep type EEG activity and atonia.

Diagnosis is made primarily by history. If an event is captured during PSG, then the EEG shows mixed patterns of REM and wakefulness with abundant alpha activity and atonia.

Differential diagnosis includes narcolepsy if EDS is present or a history of hypnic hallucinations and cataplexy can be elicited. Although daytime sleepiness is necessary to make the diagnosis of narcolepsy, sleep paralysis can also occur in other conditions that present with daytime sleepiness such as sleep deprivation, sleep-related breathing disorder and idiopathic hypersomnia. The same applies for hypnic hallucinations. When hypnic hallucinations occur together with sleep paralysis and daytime sleepiness, narcolepsy is highly likely, although the three symptoms can occur in association in severe sleep deprivation due to insufficient sleep or sleep apnea and rarely even in idiopathic hypersomnia. The diagnosis of narcolepsy can be made if there is history of unequivocal cataplexy or by doing PSG or a multiple sleep latency test (MSLT) and documenting a mean sleep latency of less than 8 minutes with two or more sleep-onset REM periods after a normal full night's sleep. Cataplexy tends to occur during the wake period and is triggered by a specific emotion.

Atonic seizures can also mimic cataplexy or sleep paralysis, but they tend to occur during wakefulness and are associated with characteristic EEG abnormalities.

Drop attacks due to ischemia in the posterior cerebral circulation are not related to the sleep/wake transition and are accompanied by dizziness, mental cloudiness and alteration of consciousness. Other conditions that are on the differential diagnosis include hypokalemic periodic paralysis, catatonia and conversion disorder. The first is much longer-lasting than sleep paralysis, often continuing for hours or days and is associated with low serum potassium levels; it has no correlation with sleep/wake transition periods. The latter two have specific psychiatric symptom characteristics for each condition and do not necessarily happen in the sleep/wake zone. It is critical to be absolutely sure before diagnosing someone with sleep paralysis with a conversion disorder, especially as dramatic and unusual symptoms can accompany the periods of sleep paralysis.

In general, patients with frequent episodes of sleep paralysis learn that the episodes are brief, benign and reversible and have no serious sequelae. This knowledge, however, may not diminish the discomfort, the subjective shortness of breath or the sense of fear that one feels during it. Although reassurance is important in isolated sleep paralysis, treatment may be required for the reasons mentioned above.

Avoiding sleep deprivation, advising good sleep hygiene, and treating jet lag syndrome and to some degree shift work syndrome can help prevent these episodes from happening. It is also important to treat underlying and co-morbid conditions, not only narcolepsy but others such as multiple sclerosis, post-traumatic stress disorder (PTSD), social phobia, panic disorder and anxiety in general. It is also important to be aware of the medicolegal and forensic implications of recurrent sleep paralysis, especially when occurring concomitantly with hypnic hallucinations, because these are sometimes misinterpreted as threatening intruders, repressed childhood memories of sexual abuse or alien abductions. Cultural variations also play a role in how a patient interprets these experiences.

When medical treatment is necessary, the first line of drugs is tricyclic antidepressants, followed by the selective serotonin reuptake inhibitors (SSRIs) and selective norepinephrine reuptake inhibitors (SNRIs). Clomipramine, imipramine or desmethylimipramine at a dose of 25–50 mg taken orally 1 hour before bedtime are very effective; also effective are protriptyline 2–10 mg, fluoxetine 10–30 mg, viloxazine 25–50 mg and femoxetine 100–150 mg.

Pearls and gold

Isolated paralysis most often occurs when awakening; this is the postdormital or hypnopompic type. The familial and sleep paralyses associated with narcolepsy tend to occur more frequently while falling asleep; this is the predormital or hypnagogic type.

Episodes occur more frequently in supine sleepers and those who experience it at the beginning and middle of the night, rather than the end of the night.

Although there is a subjective sense of shortness of breath, respiratory muscles are spared.

The first line of pharmacological treatment is tricyclic antidepressants, followed by SSRIs and SNRIs.

SUGGESTED READING

HISTORICAL

Mitchell SW. On some of the disorders of sleep. *Virginia Med Monthly* 1876; **2**: 769–81.

REVIEW

Sandyk R. Resolution of sleep paralysis by weak electromagnetic fields in a patient with multiple sclerosis. *Int J Neurosci* 1997; **90**: 145–57.

GENERAL

AASM (American Academy of Sleep Medicine). *International Classification of Sleep Disorders*, 2nd edn.: *Diagnostic and Coding Manual*. Westchester, Illinois: American Academy of Sleep Medicine, 2005.

Awadalla A, Al-Fayez G, Harville M, *et al*. Comparative prevalence of isolated sleep paralysis in Kuwaiti, Sudanese, and American college students. *Psychol Rep* 2004; **95**: 317–22.

Cheyne JA. Sleep paralysis episode frequency and number, types, and structure of associated hallucinations. *J Sleep Res* 2005; **14**: 319–24.

de Jong JT. Cultural variation in the clinical presentation of sleep paralysis. *Transcult Psychiatry* 2005; **42**: 78–92.

Girard TA, Cheyne JA. Timing of spontaneous sleep-paralysis episodes. *J Sleep Res* 2006; **15**: 222–9.

Mitler MM, Hajdukovic R, Erman M, Koziol JA. Narcolepsy. *J Clin Neurophysiol* 1990; **7**: 93–118.

Ohaeri JU, Awadalla A, Makanjuola VA, Ohaeri BM. Features of isolated sleep paralysis among Nigerians. *East Afr Med J* 2004; **81**: 509–19.

Case 12

Nightmares and numbness in the right arm

Philip Cherian, Elizabeth Budman and Antonio Culebras

Clinical history

A 27-year-old man was admitted to the hospital with right arm numbness that had been present for the previous 8 days. His right arm, thumb and second and third fingers had decreased sensation and tingling. He experienced more discomfort with heat, for example taking a hot shower, and he felt better in the cold. The patient reported visual problems that made reading difficult, also exacerbated by heat. There was a significant past history of excessive daytime sleepiness (EDS), night terrors, hypnagogic and hypnopompic hallucinations, hypnopompic sleep paralysis, and sleepwalking and sleeptalking since the age of 13 years.

There was also a past medical history of restless legs syndrome (RLS), sinus tachycardia and risky sexual behaviors. He was taking ropinirole, zolpidem and lorazepam for the various sleep problems. The patient worked as a night nurse. He smoked half a packet of cigarettes per day and drank five to six beers on two to three nights a week.

Examination

His vital signs were normal. There was mild expiratory wheezing at the bases bilaterally related to an upper respiratory infection. Visual acuity was 20/20 at 6 feet bilaterally. There was reduced sensation to light touch, pinprick and vibration in the right upper extremity in C6–C7 distribution. Mild asymmetry of patellar reflexes was noted, with the left being more prominent. A CT scan of the head showed a non-specific small area of hypoattenuation in the left frontal lobe adjacent to the left lateral ventricle. An MRI of the brain showed multiple small hyperintense lesions in white matter throughout both cerebral hemispheres and the brainstem. Some of the lesions involved subcortical regions and were suggestive of demyelination. The MRI of the cervical spine showed lesions in the cervical cord, one of them enhancing after administration of gadolinium.

Case Studies in Sleep Neurology: Common and Uncommon Presentations, ed. A. Culebras. Published by Cambridge University Press. © Cambridge University Press 2010.

His serum was negative for HIV antibody and CSF analysis and protein electro-phoresis were normal.

Special studies

An overnight sleep study followed by a multiple sleep latency test (MSLT) revealed REM sleep without atonia and abundant myoclonic jerks in REM sleep. Nocturnal REM sleep latency was mildly reduced (76 minutes). The MSLT showed mild EDS (mean sleep latency for four segments, 7.4 minutes) without the presence of REM sleep in nap segments. Overall, the study showed abnormalities of REM sleep without evidence of narcolepsy.

Question

Are the sleep alterations related to the brain lesions?

Results of studies

A diagnosis of demyelinating disorder was considered likely based on the MRI findings characterized by multiple scattered lesions and T2 hyperintensities in the right thalamus, right parietal/occipital border, bilateral frontoparietal lobes and pons (Figure 12.1). Gadolinium-enhancing lesions were seen in the left frontal lobe (Figure 12.2) and in the cervical cord. Right arm numbness was interpreted as related to the acute lesion in the cervical spinal cord, although

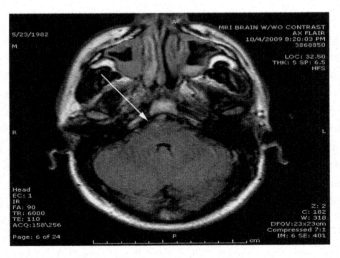

Figure 12.1 Non-enhancing small lesion in the anterior pons.

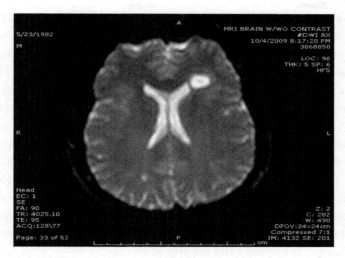

Figure 12.2 Gadolinium-enhancing lesion in the left frontal lobe suggestive of a demyelinating disorder.

other correlations could not be ruled out. Based on the results, the patient was started on interferon-β1a.

A more vexing clinical problem was posed by the relationship of a demyelinating disorder with the sleep alterations. Since the age of 13, the patient had experienced sleep behaviors characterized by sleeptalking, sleepwalking and terrors suggestive of an arousal disorder. In addition, there were episodes of sleep paralysis, and hypnopompic and hypnagogic hallucinations suggestive of REM-sleep pathology. The polysomnogram showed REM sleep without atonia, a phenomenon generally observed in correlation with REM-sleep behavior disorder (RBD). The combination of arousal disorder and RBD has been termed parasomnia overlap disorder.

Diagnosis

A diagnosis was made of probable parasomnia overlap disorder in the context of multiple sclerosis.

General remarks

Parasomnia overlap disorder is a variant of RBD. ICSD-2 (AASM, 2005) defines parasomnia overlap disorder as a combination of RBD and a disorder of arousal (sleepwalking, confusional arousal or sleep terror). Parasomnia overlap disorder, like RBD, has a male predominance with an earlier age of onset, with most cases occurring in adolescence. The term was coined by Schenck *et al.* (1997) although cases of co-existence of RBD and arousal disorder had been reported as far back as 1993 by other authors (e.g. Bokey, 1993).

Schenck and colleagues described 33 cases, all confirmed by polysomnography (PSG) to have both conditions. In their series, mean age of onset was 14.6+16.3 years with a range of 1–66 years, and 69% of patients were male. Importantly, one-third of subjects had a symptomatic form associated with neurological conditions such as multiple sclerosis, Möbius syndrome, Harlequin syndrome and traumatic brain injury, all of them suggestive of brainstem pathology. Schenck and colleagues hypothesized that neurodegenerative changes in the brainstem could affect ascending control of sleep state transitions leading to motor dyscontrol and arousals from NREM sleep and REM sleep. The treatment recommended was clonazepam, although alprazolam and carbamazepine were also suggested as favorable treatments. Parasomnia overlap disorder may have a familial incidence, but many cases are also idiopathic.

Our patient had evidence of both parasomnia overlap disorder and multiple sclerosis. It is possible that demyelinating lesions observed in the pons, albeit small and not enhancing, were responsible for the manifestations of motor dyscontrol both in NREM and REM sleep.

Lack of gadolinium enhancement in the pons suggested that the lesions were old. The accumulation of gadolinium in plaques is associated with newly active plaques and with pathologically confirmed acute inflammation in multiple sclerosis. Gadolinium enhancement is a transient phenomenon in multiple sclerosis and usually disappears after 30–40 days, rarely persisting for up to 8 weeks in acute plaques. Conventional T2-weighted MRI techniques may underestimate multiple sclerosis plaque size and thus overall plaque burden. Advanced MRI techniques such as diffusion tensor imaging and magnetic resonance spectroscopy may reveal the involvement of normal-appearing white matter in patients with multiple sclerosis.

Pearls and gold

The combination of arousal disorder and RBD defines parasomnia overlap disorder.

One-third of patients have structural or neurodegenerative lesions in the brainstem.

Parasomnia overlap disorder responds favorably to the administration of clonazepam.

Patients with parasomnia overlap disorder should be evaluated carefully to assess the presence or development of neurodegenerative conditions.

SUGGESTED READING

HISTORICAL

Bokey K. Conversion disorder revisited: severe parasomnia discovered. *Aust N Z J Psychiatry* 1993; **27**: 694.

Schenck CH, Boyd JL, Mahowald MW. A parasomnia overlap disorder involving sleepwalking, sleep terrors, and REM sleep behavior disorder in 33 polysomnographically confirmed cases. *Sleep* 1997; **20**: 972–81.

REVIEW

Mahowald MW, Schenck CH. Dissociated states of wakefulness and sleep. *Neurology* 1992; **42**: 44–52.

GENERAL

American Academy of Sleep Medicine. *International Classification of Sleep Disorders*, 2nd edn.: *Diagnostic and Coding Manual*. Westchester, Illinois: American Academy of Sleep Medicine, 2005.

Lombardi C, Vetrugn OR, Provini F, *et al.* Harlequin syndrome: an association with overlap parasomnia. *J Neurol Neurosurg Psychiatry* 2004; **75**: 341–2.

Schenck CH, Mahowald MW. Rapid eye movement sleep parasomnias. *Neurol Clin* 2005; **23**: 1107–26.

Schenkel E, Siegel JM. REM sleep without atonia after lesions of the medial medulla. *Neurosci Lett* 1989; **98**: 159–65.

Screaming at night

Maha Alattar and Bradley V. Vaughn

Clinical history

Ms. N. was a 46-year-old female with a 5-year history of distressing, unpleasant and bizarre dreams that occurred from a few times a week to once a month, depending on her stress level. The onset of these dreams was typically in the middle or latter part of the night. Being chased, violated or pinned down were common themes, and she tried to escape but a sense of immobility and fear would take over, which then triggered the screaming, waking herself up. Feeling paralyzed was a common experience during these dreams.

Each event had a storyline. In one, she was looking at a leathery and ancient-looking book that she called "the Book of Life." Once she held it, the leather cover started to move and formed a face and the book became "alive." When she opened it, the pages, revealed "very dark and disturbing secrets" such as people's future death dates. Another story involved "a bodiless entity" or ghost-like figure trying to possess her by passing through her body, but a sense of immobility and paralysis prevented her from escaping, fear took over and she woke up with a scream.

Her boyfriend, who was an eyewitness to these events, reported that she typically made a faint humming sound that quickly built up to a loud "hallow" scream, which eventually awakened both of them. She was typically drenched in sweat and her heart was beating fast.

Ms. N. reported a strong relationship between the frequency of nightmares and daily stress, such as financial difficulties and family-related issues. Although she had not been formally diagnosed with an anxiety disorder, she recounted anxiety symptoms including three panic attacks during the past 5 years. She described herself as a perfectionist.

Her bedtime and wake times were regular (11 pm and 7 am). She typically fell asleep within 30 minutes. She described her overall daily sleep quality as restful. However, nights that were dominated by a nightmare were restless and

Case Studies in Sleep Neurology: Common and Uncommon Presentations, ed. A. Culebras. Published by Cambridge University Press. © Cambridge University Press 2010.

were followed by next-day fatigue and frustration. She denied sleepwalking, symptoms of restless legs symptoms (RLS) and teeth clenching or grinding. She admitted to mild snoring. Neither she nor her boyfriend had witnessed arm or leg jerking, kicking, punching or any violent physical events.

Her medical history was unremarkable except for gastroesophageal reflux disorder, situational depression (job loss, relationship/family difficulties) and three daytime panic attacks that occurred over the past 5 years. She denied the use of tobacco and illicit drugs, but consumed one glass of wine a week. She did not take medication. She worked as a professional visual artist.

Examination

Her vital signs were normal with a blood pressure of 138/79 mmHg and a pulse of 85 bpm. A HEENT (head, ears, eyes, nose and throat) examination was normal; her Mallampati score was class 2. Her BMI was $26 \, \text{kg/m}^2$. Neurological and general examinations were normal. Her mood was appropriate and affect was normal. However, she appeared tense at times.

Special studies

Nocturnal polysomnography (PSG) was carried out, and the thyroid-stimulating hormone level in plasma was determined.

Question

What is your diagnosis?

Results of studies

Polysomnography showed a normal sleep architecture adjusted to the first-night effect. Sleep-related breathing disturbance was not noted except for occasional snoring. Periodic limb movements of sleep (PLMS) were not recorded. No nightmare episodes were reported by the patient during the study. EMG activity was normal. Thyroid-stimulating hormone level was normal.

Diagnosis

The diagnosis was nightmare disorder with primary snoring.

Follow-up

The patient was informed of her results and the diagnosis of nightmare disorder was explained. The relationship between daytime stress, anxiety and nightmares was emphasized. The treatment plan centered on addressing daily stress and anxiety. The physician discussed and instructed her on the imagery rehearsal technique (Krakow *et al.*, 1995). She was referred to a psychologist to implement stress reduction techniques and coping mechanisms in order to reduce her daytime anxiety. The patient was instructed to keep a "nightmare event calendar." During her follow-up visits, she reported a reduction in the severity and frequency of nightmares, which was also reflected in the calendar.

General remarks

Nightmare disorder is classified as a parasomnia in ICSD-2 (AASM, 2005) and is defined as "recurrent episodes of awakenings from sleep with recall of intensely disturbing dream mentation, usually involving fear or anxiety, with the patient attaining full alertness, immediate and clear recall with the associated features of subsequent delay of return to sleep or the episodes occurring in the latter half of the sleep period." A nightmare is a common human phenomenon that is reported in all ages.

Recurrent nightmares are frequent in children (20–39%) and less frequent in adults (5–8%). Nightmares are more common in women. They lead to sleep disturbance and insomnia and decreased daytime performance. Dream recall occurs in all stages of sleep but is reported more commonly during REM sleep (80% of individuals out of REM sleep versus 40% out of deep sleep). REM-sleep dreaming tends to be intensely visual with bizarre surreal details, whereas deep-sleep dreaming is vague, poorly coherent and less visual, where the theme centers around a "feeling sense" (for example, feeling the presence of a snake in the room but not actually visualizing one).

Dreams out of stages N1 and N2 are brief and simple compared with REM-sleep dreams. Some research has postulated that dreaming plays a role in memory consolidation and learning as well as emotional feedback. During REM sleep, muscle atonia gives the sensation that one cannot run away from the nightmare-associated events. The last REM-sleep episode of the night is the longest and most intense (high REM density) and tends to produce the most bizarre and vivid dreams, which are more likely to be remembered.

Nightmares also occur in patients with psychiatric illnesses such as anxiety, depression and schizophrenia, as well as in individuals with poor coping mechanisms and creative tendencies. Psychological stress plays a big role in precipitating nightmares. Nocturnal panic attacks can be difficult to differentiate from nightmares, but individuals with nocturnal panic tend also to have daytime anxiety and panic.

Nightmare disorder should be differentiated from other types of sleep and wake disorders that involve abnormal or frightening dreams. Nightmares can be part of an acute stress disorder or post-traumatic stress disorder (PTSD). Patients with PTSD re-live or experience a prior life trauma during the dream (recurrent nightmares or flashbacks); they typically awaken feeling very disturbed and develop conditioned insomnia (fear of sleeping). Post-traumatic stress disorder is commonly seen in war veterans or in victims of terrorist attacks or of severe emotional trauma (such as sexual abuse). Treatment involves intense psychotherapy and cognitive behavioral therapy (CBT) coupled at times with medications; prazosin has shown promising results.

Parasomnia disorders may present with associated nightmares and need to be differentiated from simple nightmares. Disorders of arousal, such as confusional arousals, sleepwalking and sleep terror, usually emerge out of deep sleep. REM-sleep behavior disorder (RBD), which commonly occurs in older men, is associated with REM-sleep dream enactment that includes acting out violent dreams and other behaviors such as jerking of the arms/legs, punching, screaming and falling out of bed. These patients frequently injure themselves or their bed partner. REM-sleep behavior disorder is commonly associated with neurodegenerative disorders such as Parkinson's disease or Lewy body dementia, and with narcolepsy in younger patients. Therefore, a thorough neurological evaluation is advised. Clonazepam is the treatment of choice.

Sleep or night terror (also called *pavor nocturnus*) occurs in children between the ages of 3 and 5 and is characterized by a sudden arousal from slow-wave sleep, followed by a piercing scream and an intense autonomic discharge (tachycardia, tachypnea, dilated pupils). Typically the patient's eyes are open but they do not respond to the external world because they are asleep. There is no dream recall, unlike an individual having a nightmare. Treatment is through assurance to the parents. Rarely, pharmacological intervention is needed.

Medical conditions such as nocturnal seizures, cluster or migraine headaches, cardiac disease, asthma, chronic obstructive pulmonary disease and sleep apnea need to be considered as part of the differential diagnosis of nightmare, therefore requiring further testing and evaluations. If nocturnal seizures are suspected, prolonged video-EEG monitoring might be required. Medications can alter the central nervous system neurotransmitters and cause nightmares; drugs linked to nightmares are tricyclic antidepressants, selective serotonin reuptake inhibitor (SSRIs), beta-blockers and dopamine agonists. Withdrawal from medications (benzodiazepines) or alcohol may increase the occurrence of nightmares.

Treatment of patients with nightmares requires a thorough evaluation to ensure proper diagnosis and management. Once the diagnosis of nightmare disorder is established, it is also important to consider the individual's psychological state in order to address any underlying co-morbidities such as PTSD, mood disorders or stress. There is a range of treatment options that are effective in diminishing the frequency and intensity of chronic nightmares and sleep disturbance. Nightmare-focused CBT has shown long-term benefit. During exposure and systematic desensitization, the patient is asked to recall the unpleasant dream and then reconstruct and re-live it by imagining it during the day; with repetition, the nightmare sufferer will become desensitized to the fears associated with the nightmare. Cognitive restructuring technique (imagery rehearsal technique) is slightly different in that the patient is asked to alter the nightmare theme, encouraging the subject to evoke their own special theme where the storyline or ending has a positive outcome. Patients then practice the new dream daily in the afternoon away from the sleep period. Most patients will notice diminished nightmares after 3 weeks. In addition to CBT, daytime relaxation techniques also need to be implemented. Nightmare sufferers, unfortunately, do not typically seek professional medical help. Educating primary care physicians on recognizing nightmare disorders and treatment techniques can provide rapid access to treatment. For protracted cases, a pharmacological trial of clonazepam or prazosin at bedtime might be helpful.

Pearls and gold

Recurrent nightmares are frequent in children (20–39%) and less frequent in adults (5–8%).

Nightmares are more common in women.

Dream recall occurs in all stages of sleep but is more commonly reported during REM sleep.

REM-sleep dreaming tends to be intensely visual with bizarre surreal details, whereas deep-sleep dreaming is vague, poorly coherent and less visual.

During REM sleep, muscle atonia gives the sensation that one cannot escape from the nightmare-associated events.

The last REM-sleep episode of the night is the longest and most intense (high REM density) and tends to produce the most bizarre and vivid dreams, which are more likely to be remembered.

Drugs linked to nightmares are tricyclic antidepressants, SSRIs, beta-blockers and dopamine agonists. Withdrawal from medications (benzodiazepines) or alcohol may increase nightmares.

SUGGESTED READING

HISTORICAL

Geer JH, Silverman I. Treatment of a recurrent nightmare by behavior-modification procedures: a case study. *J Abnorm Psychol* 1967; **72**: 188–90.

REVIEW

Lancee J, Spoormaker VI, Krakow B, van den Bout J. A systematic review of cognitive-behavioral treatment for nightmares: toward a well-established treatment. *J Clin Sleep Med* 2008; **4**: 475–80.

GENERAL

AASM (American Academy of Sleep Medicine). *International Classification of Sleep Disorders*, 2nd edn.: *Diagnostic and Coding Manual*. Westchester, Illinois: American Academy of Sleep Medicine, 2005.

Krakow B, Kellner R, Neidhardt J, Pathak D, Lambert L. Imagery rehearsal treatment of chronic nightmares: with a thirty month follow-up. *J Behav Ther Exp Psychiatry* 1993; **24**: 325–30.

Krakow BJ, Kellner R, Pathak D, Lambert L. Imagery rehearsal treatment for chronic nightmares. *Behav Res Ther* 1995; **33**: 837–43.

Violent sleep behavior resulting in subdural hemorrhage

Mark Eric Dyken, Kyoung Bin Im and Adel K. Afifi

Clinical history

The patient was a 73-year-old man who complained of two recent violent dreams that resulted in significant injury. He reported dreaming about a man who was running: "Someone yelled, 'Stop him.' I tried." His wife stated that, immediately prior to awakening with dream recall, he leaped off the bed and sustained superficial injuries to his head and lower extremities. During another event, he struck the right side of his face on the furniture, afterwards complaining of nausea and a headache that was followed by vomiting and slight confusion.

He had 10 years of progressively more frequent and violent dream-related behaviors and complained of almost nightly dreams where: "I act them out; sometimes I hurt myself. I go through the motions of what I'm dreaming about." The patient also indicated that he would on occasions hit his wife in association with the dreams where he believed he was protecting her. The patient's wife also noted that he "flops" his legs a lot during sleep. In addition, he had recent problems with nocturnal choking that resolved after receiving antibiotics and nasal sprays for sinusitis.

His past medical history included an anterior wall myocardial infarction (16 years previously), peptic ulcer disease, sinusitis and a remote history of tuberculosis (successfully treated with isoniazid). Surgeries included herniorrhaphy, carpal tunnel repair and a transurethral resection of the prostate for prostatitis. He discontinued a 40–60 pack a year history of tobacco use at the time of his myocardial infarction, and used alcohol infrequently. The patient's only medication was ranitidine 150 mg per day. The family history was positive for myocardial infarction in the patient's father.

Examination

The patient's vital signs included a blood pressure of 132/65 mmHg and a heart rate of 68 bpm, and his BMI was 29.0 kg/m². With regard to general appearance, right infraorbital edema was noted in association with hematoma (Figure 14.1).

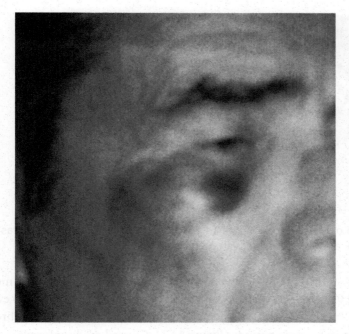

Figure 14.1 The patient at the time of his initial examination had evidence of superficial injury sustained to the right maxillary region from a reported episode of violent sleep-related behavior. (Reproduced with permission from Dyken *et al.*, 1995).

There was some oropharyngeal tissue redundancy with a Mallampati score of class 2. The patient was alert and oriented to person, place and time, and the neurological examination was otherwise unremarkable without focal findings.

Special studies

Given the recent head trauma, an MRI scan of the brain and brainstem was performed to rule out any lesion that might have contributed to or resulted from the nocturnal trauma. Standard polysomnography (PSG) using split-screen video-EEG analysis was carried out.

Question

What is your diagnosis and prognosis?

Results of studies

The MRI scan revealed a right subdural hematoma without mass effect (which subsequently resolved within 9 months), and a few small 2–3 mm foci of deep white matter changes suggesting atherosclerotic microangiopathy (Figure 14.2).

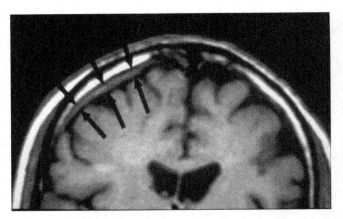

Figure 14.2 A brain MRI of the patient in Figure 14.1 revealed a subdural hemorrhage, as outlined by the black arrows. (Modified with permission from Dyken *et al.*, 1995).

The PSG study revealed significant periodic limb movements (with a movement index of 52.0 events per hour and a movement-arousal index of only 3.0 events per hour). There was an unusual increase in phasic limb movements throughout most of the REM-sleep periods (Figure 14.3). Clinical or electrographic evidence of sleep apnea or seizure activity was not identified. During one REM-sleep episode, the patient suddenly exhibited explosive running movements, after which he awoke, and in an alert and coherent manner spontaneously reported "one of them dreams – I was chasing cattle" (it should be noted that the patient farmed cattle for a living).

Follow-up

The patient was subsequently treated with clonazepam 1.0 mg every evening before sleep, with complete resolution of all violent dream-related behaviors over the following year. Nevertheless, over the next 8 years, the patient's family reported that he had a slow but progressive decline in memory and overall cognition, in association with a shuffling gait. A formal neurocognitive assessment revealed mild-to-moderate dementia with a substantial motor component. A follow-up assessment by a movement disorders specialist led to the diagnosis of Parkinson's disease. His examination at that time revealed deficits in attention and remote memory but a normal fund of knowledge, with bradykinesia, cogwheel rigidity, decreased postural reflexes and a positive palmomental reflex. A combination of levodopa/carbidopa 25/100 mg three times a day was started. Later, the patient developed symptoms and signs typically associated with the treatment and progression of Parkinson's disease, respectively: daytime hallucinations

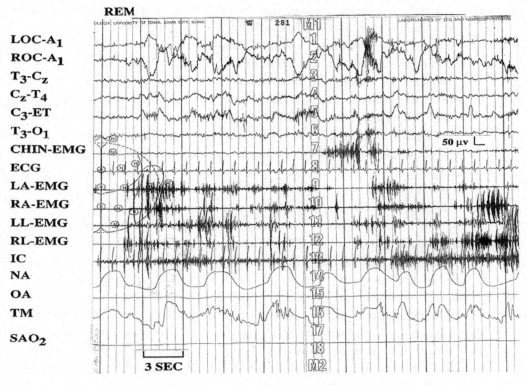

Figure 14.3 The patient's PSG tracing revealed an unusually high level of EMG augmentation during REM sleep. LOC, left outer canthus; ROC, right outer canthus; T, temporal; C, central; ET, ears tied; O, occipital; LA, left arm; RA, right arm; RL, right leg; IC, intercostal EMG; NA, nasal airflow; OA, oral airflow; TM, thoracic movement. (Reproduced with permission from Figure 17 in Dyken *et al.*, 2001).

and falls, for which he eventually required 24-hour supervision in a care center. During the patient's last visit to a physician, his complaints of progressive sleepiness led to the scheduling of a PSG to address the possibility of obstructive sleep apnea (OSA); this appointment was never kept as the patient passed away in the care facility from non-specified reasons.

Diagnosis and treatment

The patient's history and PSG analysis are classical for, and diagnostic of, REM-sleep behavior disorder (RBD), which is defined in ICSD-2 (AASM, 2005) as a parasomnia associated with REM sleep. It generally occurs while the patient is in REM sleep and is associated with violent, directed behavior that is followed by the spontaneous, non-prompted report of a detailed dream corresponding with the observed movements (isomorphism).

Up to 77.1% of patients present with mild to moderate sleep-related injuries, including bruises, lacerations, dislocations and fractures, and on rare occasions serious injuries, which have included bilateral subdural hemorrhages.

REM-sleep behavior disorder was first described in 1985, and is associated with violent behaviors arising from REM sleep (normally a state of relative paralysis). The diagnosis requires a history of potentially harmful sleep-related body movements associated with REM-sleep dreams. In the idiopathic form (not related to injury or drugs), the estimated prevalence in the general population is 0.38–0.8% (0.5% in the elderly).

Although patients may only experience a major episode once every few weeks, and PSG may only capture characteristic behaviors in 8%, PSG has still proven to be a valuable diagnostic tool. ICSD-2 criteria for defining RBD with PSG demand the presence of REM sleep without atonia. Although not a diagnostic criterion, RBD is also associated with periodic limb movements of sleep (PLMS) in up to 75% of patients; nevertheless, in RBD these movements are not frequently associated with many frank arousals.

Experts indicate that specific therapy for RBD in patients with Parkinson's disease is the same as for those with idiopathic RBD. Although RBD may become worse with the progression of Parkinson's disease, the RBD can on occasion resolve spontaneously. It has been reported that clonazepam successfully controls RBD in up to 90% of patients, without major complications with regard to drug tolerance or medication abuse. The administration of 0.5–1.0 mg usually leads to a significant reduction in the unwanted behaviors within 1–7 days. Taking the medicine approximately 2 hours prior to the desired bedtime may also help to address any underlying problems with sleep-onset insomnia that may be related to PLMS, while helping to reduce the risk of an early morning sedative hang-over effect.

The efficacy of clonazepam is hypothesized to be due to a serotonergic effect, as lesion studies of the raphe nucleus (which utilizes serotonin as a neurotransmitter) lead to an increase in REM phasic activity. The effect may be due to inhibition of locomotor systems rather than brainstem centers associated with atonia, as the PSG pattern of REM sleep without atonia generally persists despite successful treatment. Other medications that have been reported to have variable efficacy include melatonin, tricyclic antidepressants (desipramine), levodopa, pramipexole, carbamazepine, gabapentin, monoamine oxidase inhibitors, donepezil and clonidine. In Parkinson's disease, pallidotomy has anecdotally been reported to be effective in treating RBD, while bilateral subthalamic stimulation has not.

Additional care to protect the bedroom environment should also be taken, with recommendations that include placing the mattress on the floor, removing sharp or potentially dangerous objects from the bedroom and protecting the patient from the glass associated with the window area, and possibly utilizing a ground-level room should there be a possibility of falling (or jumping) through the window.

Parkinson's disease is a progressive neurodegenerative disorder that potentially affects the basic sleep/wake mechanisms located throughout the brain and brainstem. Degeneration affecting the gamma-aminobutyric acid (GABA) "sleep switch" located in the ventrolateral preoptic nucleus of the hypothalamus, or the monoaminergic waking centers (the histaminergic tuberomammillary nucleus, the serotonergic dorsal raphe and the noradrenergic locus coeruleus) can respectively lead to the very common complaints of insomnia and sleepiness. In such cases, the judicious utilization of GABA-ergic medications for insomnia and/or stimulants for sleepiness might be considered for use on an off-label basis.

In Parkinson's disease, the degenerative process may affect brainstem respiratory centers, as obstructive, central and hypoventilatory sleep-related breathing disorders have been reported with some frequency. Normal involuntary breathing is largely governed by a medullary respiratory center: the dorsal respiratory group and the ventral respiratory group. Central sleep apnea has been documented in humans after stroke of the solitary tract nucleus, and injury to the rostral ventral respiratory group has been used to explain OSA following stroke; as such, neural degeneration in these areas in Parkinson's disease might also lead to sleep-related breathing disorders. In addition, parasomnias can emerge in close association with OSA when cerebral anoxic attacks lead to violent RBD-like behavior.

Violent dream-related behaviors have also been reported in the psychiatric disorders, post-traumatic stress disorder (PTSD), somnambulism, night terrors, dream interruption insomnia, sleep apnea and seizures in sleep. Polysomnography-documented REM sleep without atonia has been associated with narcolepsy, drug use and post-traumatic stress, while PSG-documented excessive movements in sleep have been reported with seizures, paroxysmal nocturnal dystonia, somnambulism, night terrors, psychiatric conditions (such as dissociative states, malingering, PTSD and nocturnal panic attacks) and sleep drunkenness (behavioral responses to arousals induced by disorders such as OSA and possibly severe PLMS).

General remarks

REM-sleep behavior disorder may be the initial manifestation of a neurodegenerative disorder, especially the synucleinopathies, including Parkinson's disease,

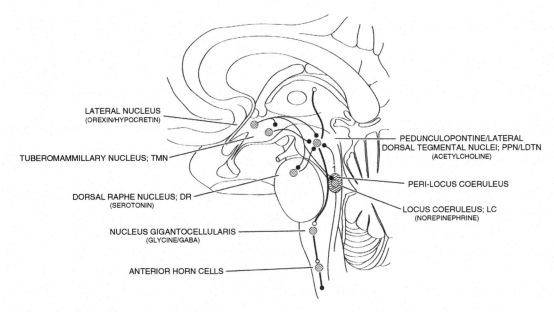

LATERAL NUCLEUS
(OREXIN/HYPOCRETIN)

PEDUNCULOPONTINE/LATERAL
DORSAL TEGMENTAL NUCLEI; PPN/LDTN
(ACETYLCHOLINE)

TUBEROMAMMILLARY NUCLEUS; TMN

PERI-LOCUS COERULEUS

DORSAL RAPHE NUCLEUS; DR
(SEROTONIN)

LOCUS COERULEUS; LC
(NOREPINEPHRINE)

NUCLEUS GIGANTOCELLULARIS
(GLYCINE/GABA)

ANTERIOR HORN CELLS

Figure 14.4 The brain and brainstem in the parasagittal plane showing the basic proposed mechanism and structures involved in generation of REM-sleep violent behaviors in RBD. In REM sleep, there is a loss of wake-promoting effects from orexin (hypocretin) cells in the lateral nucleus of the hypothalamus, the tuberomammillary nucleus, the dorsal pontine raphe nucleus, the locus coeruleus and the pedunculopontine/lateral dorsal tegmental nucleus (PPN/LDTN). This leaves cholinergic "REM-sleep on" related cells in the PPN/LDTN uninhibited, allowing stimulation of the nucleus gigantocellularis, which then hyperpolarizes anterior horn cells in the spinal cord, resulting in atonia. In RBD, degeneration of cells in the peri-locus coeruleus area is believed to disrupt the descending tracts that would normally lead to atonia, thus allowing violent behaviors during REM/dreaming sleep. Open circles, neurons activated during REM sleep; closed circles, neurons inactivated during REM sleep. (Modified with permission from Figure 1 in Dyken & Yamada, 2005).

multiple system atrophy and dementia with Lewy body disease. Thirty-three percent of patients with newly diagnosed Parkinson's disease and 90% with multiple system atrophy have been reported to have RBD. Approximately 66% of men over 50 years with idiopathic RBD develop Parkinsonism within 13 years of diagnosis.

Normal REM sleep results from uninhibited "REM-sleep on" cells that reside in the midbrain in the pedunculopontine lateral dorsal tegmental nuclear complex (Figure 14.4). Rostrally directed neurons project to several thalamic nuclei with cortical relays, while caudal projections stimulate motor activity centers in the peri-locus coeruleus region, which subsequently (through the lateral tegmento-reticular tract) activate the nucleus gigantocellularis located in the medulla. The nucleus gigantocellularis, via the ventrolateral reticulospinal tract, leads to atonia through glycine/GABA inhibition of alpha motor neurons.

Animal models suggest that, in neurodegenerative disorders such as Parkinson's disease, there can be an interruption of the REM sleep/atonia pathway and/or disinhibition of brainstem motor pattern generators, predisposing to RBD. Animal studies and human stroke reports have suggested that there may be a co-localization of atonia and locomotor systems in regions medial to the locus coeruleus (the sublateral dorsal nucleus). In addition, the pedunculopontine nucleus (in the rostral pons-caudal midbrain) lies in an area from which walking movements can be elicited (a locomotor center). A lesion in the peri-locus coeruleus region, or excessive stimulation from the pedunculopontine nucleus, could both hypothetically lead to RBD.

In Parkinson's disease, neural degeneration is thought to begin in the lower brainstem. Neuronal intrusion of Lewy bodies (the neuropathological marker of Parkinson's disease) and accumulations of insoluble α-synclein protein into cells of the peri-locus region could lead to RBD in patients who have active or even pre-clinical Parkinson's disease.

The clinical or pathophysiological subtypes of RBD include subclinical (preclinical) RBD, parasomnia overlap disorder and *status dissociatus*. Subclinical RBD occurs in patients without a clinical history of RBD but with a PSG study that shows REM sleep without atonia. It has been estimated that at least 25% of these patients will eventually develop RBD. Parasomnia overlap disorder occurs when the diagnosis of RBD occurs in combination with a disorder of arousal (confusional arousal, sleepwalking or sleep terrors). *Status dissociatus* is an extreme form of RBD in which a significant medical condition is always present, and there is a breakdown in the PSG pattern to where no identifiable sleep stages can be identified (possibly seen in end-stage Parkinson's disease).

Pearls and gold

RBD is a dream-driven event that can lead to serious injuries affecting the patient and the bed partner.

A high percentage of RBD patients develop Parkinson's disease.

Polysomnography generally shows REM sleep without atonia.

Clonazepam at bedtime is the treatment of choice.

SUGGESTED READING

HISTORICAL

Schenck CH, Bundlie SR, Mahowald MW. Human REM sleep chronic behavior disorders: a new category of parasomnia. *Sleep Res* 1985; **14**: 208.

REVIEWS

Afifi AK, Bergman RA. Reticular formation, wakefulness, and sleep. In: Afifi AK, Bergman RA, eds. *Functional Neuroanatomy, Text and Atlas*, 2nd edn. New York: McGraw-Hill, 2005, 398–406.

Dyken ME, Yamada T, Lin-Dyken DC. Polysomnographic assessment of spells in sleep: nocturnal seizures versus parasomnias. *Semin Neurol* 2001; **21**: 377–90.

Mahowald MW, Schenck CH. REM sleep parasomnias. In: Kryger MH, Roth T, Dement WC, eds. *Principles and Practice of Sleep Medicine*, 4th edn. Philadelphia: Elsevier Saunders, 2005; 897–916.

GENERAL

AASM (American Academy of Sleep Medicine). *International Classification of Sleep Disorders*, 2nd edn.: *Diagnostic and Coding Manual*. Westchester, Illinois: American Academy of Sleep Medicine, 2005.

Culebras A, Moore JT. Magnetic resonance findings in REM sleep behavior disorder. *Neurology* 1989; **39**: 1519–23.

Dyken ME, Im KB. Sleep-disordered breathing and stroke. In: Silber MH, ed. *Sleep Medicine Clinics*, Vol. 3: *Neurologic Disorders and Sleep*. Philadelphia: Elsevier Saunders, 2008; 361–76.

Dyken ME, Yamada T. Narcolepsy and disorders of excessive somnolence. *Prim Care* 2005; **32**: 389–413.

Dyken ME, Lin-Dyken DC, Seaba P, *et al.* Violent sleep-related behavior leading to subdural hemorrhage. *Arch Neurol* 1995; **52**: 318–21.

Dyken ME, Yamada T, Ali Moshin. Treatment of hypersomnias. In: Kushida CA, ed. *Handbook of Sleep Disorders*, 2nd edn. New York: Informa, 2009; 299–320.

Trenkwalder, C. Parkinsonism. In: Kryger MH, Roth T, Dement WC, eds. *Principles and Practice of Sleep Medicine*, 4th edn. Philadelphia: Elsevier Saunders, 2005; 801–10.

Xi Z, Luning W. REM sleep behavior disorder in a patient with pontine stroke. *Sleep Medicine* 2009; **10**: 143–6.

B. Arousal disorders

Case 15

Amnestic nocturnal behavior

Michael J. Howell and Carlos H. Schenck

Clinical history

A 38-year-old female patient, together with her husband of 10 years, presented to a university sleep disorders center to address amnestic nocturnal behavior. The patient described frequent sleepwalking as a child, which nearly resolved in adolescence with subsequent rare episodes (once to twice a decade) until 2005. At that time, her husband noted a surge in various night-time behaviors for which she claimed to have only minimal recall. This was associated with a new diagnosis of hepatitis B and subsequent sleep-initiation difficulties.

After the onset of hepatitis, the episodes increased in frequency to once or twice a week. The behaviors varied in duration and character but typically occurred during the first half of the sleep period. Most commonly, they consisted of agitated awakenings followed by prolonged nonsensical conversations. In particular, the husband claimed that she would verbally berate him for up to an hour at a time. This was atypical, as they both described a respectful, friendly, daytime relationship. Frequently, these episodes were associated with seemingly purposeless ambulation and activity. Examples included moving furniture to non-functional locations and bringing a bicycle into the living room. Attempts by her husband to awaken her often resulted in more assaultive language. Conversely, the husband also described amnestic episodes where she would initiate sexual intercourse. While the patient had little or no recall of these behaviors, she did not doubt that they occurred as her husband described.

The patient also engaged in frequent nocturnal binge eating and occasional dangerous behaviors. For example, she had placed various food contents into a mixer, subsequently blended them together and drank the contents. Furthermore, she would occasionally include alcohol (vodka) in these liquid meals and swallow them in a careless manner, often to the bewilderment of her husband. Surprisingly, the patient claimed she would then awaken refreshed, neither feeling intoxicated or in withdrawal. She speculated that a 10 kg weight gain was related

Case Studies in Sleep Neurology: Common and Uncommon Presentations, ed. A. Culebras. Published by Cambridge University Press. © Cambridge University Press 2010.

to these nocturnal eating binges as she had not changed her daytime caloric intake or her exercise routine. Alarmingly, there had been at least three episodes where she had gradually become aware that she was driving her car. On one occasion, she did not realize what had happened until she returned home and saw a receipt indicating that she had bought gas and a lottery ticket.

Besides the diagnosis of hepatitis B, the patient was not aware of any medical or pharmacological association with the amnestic behavior.

The patient shared a bed with her husband and typically attempted to initiate sleep at approximately 10 pm. The television was often on for the duration of the evening. Since the time of diagnosis with hepatitis B, she had had difficulty with sleep initiation. This complaint, interpreted as insomnia, had been treated with nightly zolpidem 5 mg. However, a careful history revealed that she did not suffer from insomnia. In particular, she described her inability to fall asleep being secondary to an overwhelming feeling of restlessness in her lower extremities, which worsened with quiescence and was temporarily relieved with movement. It was her impression that if these sensations were eliminated, she would not have sleep initiation difficulties. Once asleep, her husband noticed frequent leg movements throughout the night.

The patient also described daytime memory lapses. She often felt tired and confused for the first 2 hours after waking up. During this time, she had episodes of partially amnestic eccentric behavior such as placing her keys and cell phone in the refrigerator. Her primary care provider was especially concerned about whether these behaviors indicated seizures or an impending dementing illness. Despite these concerns, the patient functioned well as an executive in a large company and regularly participated in athletic activities.

Medications included levocetirizine, sertraline, loratadine, adefovir and zolpidem. Her past medical/surgical history revealed hepatitis B, major depressive disorder (in remission), childhood tonsiladenoidectomy and seasonal allergies. Her social history revealed that the patient was a college graduate who described herself as religious, happily married and professionally successful. There were loaded firearms in the house. She was adopted as a child from Honduras and raised in Minnesota. There were no health records of her biological relatives.

Examination

She was a friendly, non-dysmorphic patient who cooperated throughout the examination. Her vital signs were normal except for a BMI of 26 kg/m^2 (borderline overweight range) and borderline systolic hypertension.

A neurological specialty examination was essentially normal. Specifically, she was right-handed, alert, oriented, with excellent immediate and delayed recall of three words. Her language, calculation and executive testing revealed no abnormality. Her mood and affect were bright and congruent. In particular, there was no evidence on examination of subtle changes suggestive of a dementing illness or a parkinsonian syndrome.

Special studies

An EEG carried out in 2005 and 2009 demonstrated normal awake and drowsy responses. An MRI carried out in 2009 showed normal brain. Neuropsychological testing in 2009 revealed average or above average memory, as well as normal language, executive abilities, calculation skills and personality measures. Importantly, we were uncertain at what time of day the testing was conducted and whether she had taken zolpidem the previous evening.

The ferritin level in blood was 52 ng/ml (borderline low).

Question

What is your diagnosis?

Results of studies

Polysomnography (PSG) showed that sleep was initiated without a sedative-hypnotic. She had normal sleep architecture without any evidence of increased slow-wave sleep. Sleep-disordered breathing was not noted (apnea–hypopnea index [AHI] <1 event per hour); however, frequent periodic leg movements were identified (~40 events per hour). A full seizure montage did not demonstrate clinical or EEG evidence of seizure activity. There was no evidence for either phasic or tonic elevation of EMG tone during REM sleep.

Diagnosis

A diagnosis was made of mixed NREM parasomnia characterized by confusional arousals, sleepwalking (with sleepdriving), sleep-related eating disorder, and sexsomnia exacerbated by zolpidem. She also had restless legs syndrome (RLS).

Follow-up

The following treatment recommendations were made:

- Discontinue zolpidem and avoid other sedative agents such as alcohol.
- Treat sleep initiation failure with a dopaminergic agonist for RLS.
- If nocturnal eating persists, consider topiramate therapy.

- Recommend the patient avoid sleep deprivation.
- Address environmental safety issues such as the removal of firearms.

General remarks

Sedative-hypnotic-induced complex sleep behaviors represent an incomplete arousal of the brain from NREM sleep. Short confusional arousals, typically lasting less than 1 minute, are within the spectrum of normal sleep behavior. These activities represent a distortion of the normally sharp rise to wakefulness from a state of amnesia and diminished executive function during slow-wave sleep. They are often terminated by a more complete arousal. By suppressing arousal, benzodiazepine receptor agonists (BRAs), such as zolpidem, promote prolonged confusional arousals with complex behaviors. Furthermore, these agents selectively inhibit memory and executive function as agonists of the gamma-aminobutyric acid A (GABA$_A$) receptor. This promotes atypical behavior without recall of events. As in this case, the behavior is often primitive (aggression, binge eating, impulsive sexual activity), from diminished frontal lobe activity. These episodes are common side effects of many sedative-hypnotics and are not limited to BRAs. Responding to multiple cases of dangerous sleepwalking, the FDA has requested a new safety warning on all hypnosedatives.

This case illustrates the importance of correctly identifying the etiology of sleep initiation failure. Zolpidem, a medication with an indication for insomnia, was inappropriately prescribed for RLS, a distinct condition that superficially resembles insomnia. In our experience, most cases of sedative-hypnotic-induced complex behaviors are actually afflicted with either RLS or a circadian rhythm disorder such as delayed sleep phase syndrome. Furthermore, even well-educated patients may miss the association between the sedative-hypnotic medication and nocturnal behaviors. In this case, the patient's behaviors worsened soon after she was prescribed zolpidem. The patient attributed her symptoms to psychological stress stemming from the new diagnosis of hepatitis B. Restless legs syndrome is common in patients with chronic hepatic disease (62% in one series) and should be considered when sleep initiation difficulties arise.

Based on the dramatic nature of the clinical history, these patients often undergo extensive neuropsychological testing. This case was complicated by morning episodes that occurred after morning arousal (see below). An accurate diagnosis requires a careful history with a particular focus on co-existing sleep disorders and medication use. Polysomnographic evaluation is frequently necessary to rule out other sleep disorders that interrupt consolidated sleep, such as obstructive sleep apnea (OSA), periodic limb movement disorder (PLMD) and also nocturnal seizures that can manifest with bizarre, recurrent nocturnal behaviors.

This case also illustrates some interesting and dangerous parasomnia subtypes. Sleep-related eating disorder (SRED) represents a break from the sleep fasting state. It is characterized by recurrent episodes of eating after an arousal from night-time sleep with adverse consequences. Patients may binge eat large amounts of atypical foods, resulting in various medical consequences. These include weight gain and occasionally exacerbation of conditions such as diabetes and OSA. Zolpidem in particular is known to precipitate SRED, and in some cases may convert patients with occasional conscious nocturnal eating, as in this patient, to amnestic SRED. Furthermore, this case also illustrates confusional arousals and somnambulistic sexual behavior. This phenomenon, called sexsomnia, frequently arises in the setting of other sleepwalking behaviors and sedative medications. The amnestic activity is often different from wakeful sexual activity and is thus consistent with the loss of frontal lobe inhibition characteristic of other sleepwalking behaviors. Those afflicted often go undiagnosed, but recent forensic cases have illustrated their clinical relevance. Finally, sleepdriving, although uncommon, is a dangerous situation that requires immediate intervention. Sleepdriving is unusual in the absence of sedative medications, as the amnesia of idiopathic sleepwalking is typically of shorter duration. Considering the risk to the patient and the public, we recommend that, for those with complex sleep-related behaviors, car keys be hidden by a friend or family member and that the bedroom door is alarmed.

Many cases of BRA-induced sleepwalking behaviors are associated with supratherapeutic dosing. For example, zolpidem-induced SRED is often noted with doses higher than 10 mg. That was not noted in this case, as the patient experienced these behaviors with low dosing (5 mg). We speculate that this patient's hepatitis B may have interfered with the metabolism of zolpidem (hepatic enzyme CYP3A4).

An atypical finding in this case was the amnestic daytime episodes occurring in the morning. This worrisome behavior prompted a work-up for seizure. These episodes always occurred within the first 2 hours of attempted awakening from sleep and in association with profound sleepiness, thus comprising a form of "sleep inertia." Considering the timing and nature of these episodes, as well as the negative seizure work-up, we concluded that they most likely represented a lingering medication side effect. Importantly, these events resolved after the patient discontinued the zolpidem.

As with this case, most NREM parasomnias are effectively treated by removal of an offending agent or treatment of co-existing sleep disorders. Moreover, it is important to address issues regarding sleep hygiene such as avoiding sleep deprivation and/or irregular sleep hours and minimizing or avoiding the use of alcohol in the evening, as well as removing exogenous stimulation such as television that may fragment sleep and exacerbate dream mentation.

Bedroom safety is of critical importance considering the sporadic and relapsing nature of parasomnias. In particular, it is important to remove firearms from the house as well as placing door alarms to help wake the patient and alert family members.

In cases that are not responsive to the removal of offending agents, sleep hygiene adjustments or treatment of underlying sleep disorders, medications may be effective. Most NREM parasomnias are effectively treated with clonazepam, which, paradoxically, although a benzodiazepine, suppresses nocturnal behavior. Sleep-related eating disorder in isolation is most commonly treated with the anti-seizure medication topiramate at bedtime. Pramipexole, an anti-RLS agent, is often effective in cases of SRED and co-existent RLS.

This patient's episodes nearly resolved after discontinuing zolpidem. After 3 months, the patient and her spouse described only one confusional arousal that was relatively short-lived, did not involve sleepwalking and occurred in the setting of sleep deprivation. Furthermore, a therapeutic trial of pramipexole 1 hour prior to bedtime quickly resolved the patient's RLS and PLMD, as described in her husband's report. As the patient's borderline iron deficiency may have been contributing to her RLS, we recommended daily iron supplementation and planned to recheck ferritin levels in 6 months. Finally, we advised her to remove the television from the bedroom, have her car keys hidden and place an alarm on her bedroom door. Furthermore, we suggested that firearms should be removed from the house entirely, or at least the ammunition.

Pearls and gold

Complex sleep behaviors are uncommon; they may represent dangerous side effects of sedative-hypnotic medication, most commonly the BRAs.

In many cases of medication-induced sleepwalking, the underlying diagnosis of insomnia is incorrect. We advise clinicians to consider undiagnosed RLS or a circadian rhythm disorder, such as delayed sleep phase syndrome.

Aberrant behaviors may result in prolonged amnestic episodes involving aggressive sleeptalking, eating, driving or sexual behavior.

Elimination of the offending medication and treatment of underlying sleep disorders typically resolve the behavior.

Medications used therapeutically in idiopathic cases include clonazepam (for confusional arousals and sleepwalking), topiramate (for SRED) and pramipexole (for cases associated with RLS).

SUGGESTED READING

REVIEWS

Howell MJ, Schenck CH, Crow SJ. A review of nighttime eating disorders. *Sleep Med Rev* 2009 **13**: 23–34.

Schenck CH, Arnulf I, Mahowald MW. Sleep and sex: what can go wrong? A review of the literature on sleep related disorders of abnormal sexual behaviors and experiences. *Sleep* 2007; **30**: 683–702.

GENERAL

Andersen ML, Poyares D, Alves RSC, Skomo R, Tufik S. Sexsomnia: abnormal sexual behavior during sleep. *Brain Res Rev* 2007; **56**: 271–82.

Dolder CR, Nelson MH. Hypnosedative-induced complex behaviours: incidence, mechanisms, and management. *CNS Drugs* 2008; **22**: 1021–36.

Franco RA, Ashwanthnarayan R, Deshpandee A, *et al*. The high prevalence of restless legs syndrome in liver disease in an academic-based hepatology practice. *J Clin Sleep Med* 2008; **4**: 45–9.

Wills L, Garcia J. Parasomnias: epidemiology and management. *CNS Drugs* 2002; **16**: 803–10.

A terrified and terrifying scream

Hrayr P. Attarian

Clinical history

Mrs. A. is a 48-year-old woman who, about 1 year ago, started having episodes of sitting upright in bed, letting out a blood curdling scream and patting the bed with both hands and often going back to sleep without realizing what had happened. Rarely, she would yell loud enough to be awakened by her own voice and reported the vague memory of spiders falling on the bed. These events were initially occurring once or twice a month only at night, about 45 minutes to 1 hour after having gone to bed, but recently they had started occurring once or twice a week and even during afternoon naps. She did not complain of daytime sleepiness (Epworth Sleepiness Scale score 7/24; see Appendix) or of insomnia, but was clearly concerned about these events, especially because they disrupted her husband's sleep and were gradually becoming more frequent. She denied being told that she was a snorer or that she stopped breathing in her sleep; she also denied enuresis, nocturia or night sweats. She denied injuring herself or her husband during these spells and never got out of bed. She denied experiencing sleep paralysis or hypnic hallucinations and denied cataplexy. There had been no oral trauma and she denied achiness in the mornings. She was perimenopausal but still had regular menses and did not think the events became more frequent perimenstrually.

Coincidentally with the start of these events, her daughter had ended a short-lived marriage and moved back in with her parents bringing along her infant son. The new living arrangement had caused her mother, Mrs. A., significant psychosocial stress.

Mrs. A. also stated that she used to have night terrors as a child of 8–9 years, but they went away spontaneously after about 1 year, only occurring rarely when she was sleep deprived throughout adolescence and early adulthood. She was not on any medications and only took lisinopril for hypertension. She denied any other health problems, and denied any head trauma, perinatal injury, febrile

Case Studies in Sleep Neurology: Common and Uncommon Presentations, ed. A. Culebras. Published by Cambridge University Press. © Cambridge University Press 2010.

seizures or any type of current or past seizures. The patient did not smoke or use tobacco, did not abuse recreational drugs, rarely drank alcohol and had a cup of coffee a day.

Her family history was significant only for sleepwalking in her brother when he was in his early adolescence, but there were no sleep terrors in any first-degree family member.

Examination

The patient was a pleasant, thin, middle-aged woman in no acute distress. The neurological and general examinations were normal.

Special studies

The specialist ordered an MRI of the brain with special thin cuts through the frontal and temporal lobes, and nocturnal polysomnography (PSG) with an additional all-night 16-channel EEG running concomitantly with the PSG.

Question

What is your diagnosis: night terrors or epileptic seizures?

Follow-up

The MRI was normal as well as the nocturnal PSG and the 7-hour EEG. The patient slept for 423 minutes and had 10% stage N1, 55% stage N2, 20% stage N3 and 15% REM sleep. She had no respiratory events and her apnea–hypopnea (AHI) index was 0 per hour with a nadir oxyhemoglobin saturation of 93% and a mean saturation of 96%. She had occasional periodic limb movements (PLMs) without arousals, with a PLM index of 4 per hour. She had one 20-minute awakening at 1 am but otherwise no sleep disruptions. The EEG showed no epileptiform abnormalities, no interhemispheric asymmetries and no electrographic seizures. She had none of her typical events on the night of testing. In order to capture typical events on video and EEG, the patient was admitted to the epilepsy monitoring unit for 48 hours.

Results of studies

Two typical and almost identical events were captured on video-EEG on two consecutive nights. With the first event, the patient sat bolt upright in bed 1 hour

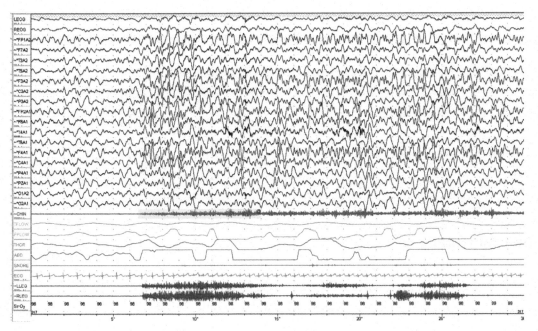

Figure 16.1 A 30-second epoch with an EEG gain of 10 μV/mm. The high frequency filter is set at 70 Hz and low-frequency filter at 1 Hz. Paper speed 30 mm/s. Note the anteriorly predominant large amplitude slow activity on EEG and the lower amplitude faster activity in the more posterior leads. Note the increase in the respiratory rate, heart rate and EMG activity. LEOG/REOG, left/right electro-oculogram; TFLOW, thermistor flow monitor; PFLOW, pressure flow monitor; THOR, thorax; ABD, abdomen; SpO₂, arterial oxyhemoglobin saturation.

after having fallen asleep; her eyes were open, she was looking around with a terrified look on her face and she let out a short series of progressively loudening screams. She simultaneously patted the bed vigorously with both hands for about 2 minutes. When awakened by the nursing staff, she became alert immediately, initially puzzled as to why she was woken up and with their question, "Are you OK?" She responded "Of course, why?" She did not know what had happened but knew she was in the hospital and was oriented to time and person. When she was told she had had a typical spell, she nodded and went back to sleep. The second event was similar, but there was only a single loud scream with similar arm movements; the event lasted less than a minute. By the time the nursing staff got into the room, she was asleep again.

During the first event, the EEG showed no epileptiform abnormalities (Figure 16.1). The anterior and middle channels showed slow activity (0.5–3 Hz) of 75–100 μV in amplitude and the posterior channels showed faster (8–9 Hz) and lower amplitude (40–50 μV) activity. There was increased muscle tone in both the chin and lower extremity channels. The respiratory rate increased from 20 to 28 breaths per minute and the heart rate increased from 60 to 95 bpm; the ECG otherwise remained normal. During the second event, the EEG and EMG channels showed the same findings, but the respiratory and heart rates did not increase as dramatically.

Diagnosis

Given these results, a diagnosis of sleep terrors or disorder of partial arousal was made.

General remarks

At the follow-up visit, the specialist gave Mrs. A. and her husband an overview of the test results, prognosis of the disorder and management. He prescribed clomipramine 25 mg at bedtime, a dose that could be increased to 50 mg if necessary. He also referred the patient to a behavioral therapist for relaxation and self-hypnosis. On the return visit, 6 weeks later, she reported a significant reduction in her events but continued to have at least one a month. She was also having dry mouth as a side effect from the clomipramine. Her medication was switched to clonazepam 0.5 mg and she was urged to follow up with the behavior therapist. Six months later, her events were all well controlled by the behavioral therapy recommendations so she was able to come off the clonazepam without recurrences.

Sleep terror, also known as night terror or *pavor nocturnus*, consists of an abrupt arousal, a sudden "blood curdling" scream or series of screams followed by incoherent vocalizations. The patients then manifest intense fear: flushing, sweating, pupillary dilation and rapid breathing, but rarely leave the bed. When they do, they usually jump out of bed and run through the house, ending in an episode of sleepwalking. Attacks usually occur during the first third of the night, but, when frequent, they could occur at any time of the night and during daytime naps. Nocturnal frontal lobe epilepsy (NFLE) is the number one differential diagnosis and must be ruled out, especially in adults. The episodes generally last between 1 and 5 minutes but sometimes may go on for as long as 15–20 minutes. The patient is unresponsive or partially responsive during the spells. As the episode ends, the patient calms down and sleep follows easily, and the episodes usually do not recur more than once per night. Recall of the episode is usually absent or limited to a single scary image, such as bugs crawling on them or being buried alive.

Sleep terror episodes can be precipitated by physical illness, especially a febrile one, or by psychological stress, sleep deprivation, forced arousals or central nervous system depressant drugs such as sedative-hypnotics, neuroleptics, minor tranquilizers, withdrawal from stimulants, and antihistamines, often in combination with each other. Although psychosocial stressors play an important role in precipitating the events, the majority of patients, both children and adults (contrary to popular belief), do not have extensive psychopathology.

According to the diagnostic criteria of ICSD-2 (AASM, 2005), the necessary features to make the diagnosis are as follows:

1. A sudden episode of terror occurs during sleep, usually initiated by a cry or a loud scream that is accompanied by autonomic and behavioral manifestations of intense fear.
2. At least one of the following features is present
   (a) Difficulty arousing the patient.
   (b) Mental confusion when awakened from an episode.
   (c) Partial or total amnesia for the events during the episode.
   (d) Dangerous or potentially dangerous behaviors.
3. The disturbance is not better explained by another sleep, medical, neurological or mental disorder, or by substance abuse or by medication side effects.

Although there is a clear familial tendency, the etiology and pathophysiology of sleep terrors remain unknown. Prevalence in prepubertal children is 1–6%, peaking around age 6 years. By age 8 years, 50% of children no longer have attacks and only 36% continue to have attacks into adolescence. In adults, the prevalence is about 1% and the majority of adults have had them as children and continued to have them throughout adolescence, often at a lower frequency. The prevalence is equal in males and females and there is no racial or cultural predilection.

The differential diagnosis includes NFLE, dissociative disorder and REM-sleep behavior disorder (RBD), especially in adults. There have been case reports of sleep terror-like activity in the setting of thalamic tumors, therefore neuroimaging is also indicated, especially when the onset is in adulthood or there is a worsening in severity and frequency.

Video-EEG monitoring is mandatory, especially if the events are frequent and/or violent, and particularly if they occur in adulthood.

EEG during an episode usually shows diffuse, hypersynchronous, rhythmic delta activity of 0.5–3 Hz in frequency and higher than 70 μV in amplitude with intermixed faster frequencies mostly in the alpha (8–12 Hz) range. This is associated with a marked increase in muscle tone, respiratory rate and heart rate.

In RBD, there is preserved muscle tone in REM sleep, no autonomic hyperactivity and intense dream recall. With epileptic phenomena, there are often epileptiform abnormalities on EEG channels during the event, and with dissociative disorders, the EEG during the event usually shows a normal awake pattern.

Safety measures to protect the patient from injury are the first line of treatment for all age groups. In children, the mainstay of treatment is eliminating precipitating causes, such as sleep deprivation, and reassurance. In adults, psychotherapy, especially stress reduction by relaxation therapy, hypnotherapy and autogenic training, can help. Pharmacotherapy includes low-dose imipramine (10–50 mg) or clomipramine (25–75 mg) at bedtime, or low-dose benzodiazepines such as clonazepam, up to 2 mg also at bedtime. There are also anecdotal reports of paroxetine, trazodone, melatonin and L-5-hydroxytryptophan being beneficial.

Pearls and gold

Sleep terror, also known as night terror or *pavor nocturnus*, consists of an abrupt arousal, with a "blood curdling" scream or series of screams, followed by incoherent vocalizations along with autonomic and behavioral manifestations of intense fear.

Attacks usually occur during the first third of the night, but when frequent, they can occur at any time of the night and during daytime naps.

Sleep terror episodes can be precipitated by physical illness, especially if febrile, or psychological stress, sleep deprivation, forced arousals or central nervous system depressant drugs.

Video-EEG monitoring is mandatory, especially if the events are frequent and/or violent, particularly if they occur in adulthood.

Safety measures to protect the patient from injury are the first line of treatment for all age groups.

SUGGESTED READING

HISTORICAL

Gastaut H, Broughton R. A clinical and polygraphic study of episodic phenomena during sleep. *Biol Psychiatry* 1965; **7**: 197–221.

Jones E. *On the Nightmare*. London: Hogarth, 1949.

REVIEW

Crisp AH. The sleepwalking/night terrors syndrome in adults. *Postgrad Med J* 1996; **72**: 599–604.

GENERAL

AASM (American Academy of Sleep Medicine). *International Classification of Sleep Disorders*, 2nd edn: *Diagnostic and Coding Manual*. Westchester, Illinois: American Academy of Sleep Medicine, 2005.

Bruni O, Ferri R, Miano S, Verrillo E. L-5-hydroxytryptophan treatment of sleep terrors in children. *Eur J Pediatr* 2004; **163**: 402–7.

Di Gennaro G, Autret A, Mascia A, *et al.* Night terrors associated with thalamic lesion. *Clin Neurophysiol* 2004; **115**: 2489–92.

Hauri PJ, Silber MH, Boeve BF. The treatment of parasomnias with hypnosis: a 5-year follow-up study. *J Clin Sleep Med* 2007; **3**: 369–73.

Hublin C, Kaprio J. Genetic aspects and genetic epidemiology of parasomnias. *Sleep Med Rev* 2003; **7**: 413–21.

Ohayon MM, Guilleminault C, Priest RG. Night terrors, sleepwalking, and confusional arousals in the general population: their frequency and relationship to other sleep and mental disorders. *J Clin Psychiatry* 1999; **60**: 268–76.

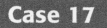
Case 17

Frequent night-time wanderings

Hrayr P. Attarian

Clinical history

Mrs. S. was a 38-year-old woman when she presented to the sleep center's outpatient clinic for evaluation of frequent sleepwalking episodes. Mrs. S. stated that since she was an adolescent she had had episodes of sleepwalking that occurred once or twice a year. About a year ago, however, her sleepwalking got significantly worse in both intensity and frequency for no reason apparent to her. She had had no change in her health or life circumstances prior to the worsening. She stated that not only was the frequency of sleepwalking almost nightly but she had ended up occasionally hurting herself by banging into objects, and once or twice she was smoking while asleep and ended up burning herself. She was very concerned and sought medical attention. She was sent to another sleep physician in her home town who started her on clonazepam. Clonazepam decreased the number of events to a certain degree but not their intensity, and she continued to have bumps and bruises due to the sleepwalking. She then followed up with her primary care physician who gradually increased the clonazepam to 3 mg a day; with this dose she had sleepwalking episodes only about twice a month, which was better than five to six times a week, but still more than they were prior to the worsening of her symptoms a year ago.

In addition to the increase in sleepwalking, she had worsening of her night-time sleep as well and worsening of her daytime alertness, especially with the increase in the clonazepam dose. To help her sleep better, eszopiclone was added to her regimen, but this only improved things modestly. She continued to have problems maintaining sleep and staying alert during the day. Her husband stated that, even with her sleepwalking episodes being reduced to twice a month, she was still sitting upright in bed multiple times a night for a few minutes, still asleep, without realizing that she had done it. Her husband stated that her sleepwalking and the sitting upright in bed tended to occur more during the first part of the night.

She went to bed between 9 and 10.30 pm, fell asleep within 15 minutes and then woke up two or three times a night to use the bathroom; she was unable to

Case Studies in Sleep Neurology: Common and Uncommon Presentations, ed. A. Culebras. Published by Cambridge University Press. © Cambridge University Press 2010.

go back to sleep for 15–30 minutes after returning to bed. She got up between 4 and 5 in the morning. In the afternoon, she took 1–2 hour naps after which she felt groggier than before. She never had a sleepwalking episode out of naps. She never woke up with oral trauma, never had enuresis and, according to her and her husband, she never had daytime seizures. During the day, she was very fatigued and sleepy. Her Epworth Sleepiness Scale score was 13 (see Appendix). She had fallen asleep behind the wheel a couple of times.

The patient denied symptoms of restless legs or observed pauses and gasps in her breathing. She denied cataplexy, sleep paralysis, hypnagogic hallucinations, waking up with heartburn or headache, choking or gasping for air.

Her past medical history was significant for panic attacks and agoraphobia, hypercholesterolemia, hypertension, asthma and stress incontinence.

She was allergic to bupropion and simvastatin and was taking enalapril, pravastatin, hydrochlorothiazide, aspirin, fenofibrate, eszopiclone, clonazepam, oxybutynin, duloxetine and albuterol.

She was a heavy smoker of 40 pack-years. She did not consume caffeine, alcohol or recreational drugs. She was married with three children and did not work outside the house. She had no significant family history for sleep disorders.

Examination

She was a pleasant, obese, young woman in no acute distress. The enurological examination was normal. Height was 165 cm, weight 85.5 kg and BMI 31.4 kg/m^2. Her vital signs were otherwise normal. A general examination was also normal.

Special studies

The specialist ordered polysomnography (PSG) with video-EEG monitoring, a pressure transducer, thermistor, chest and abdomen effort belts, electro-oculogram, chin and lower extremity EMG and oximetry. The PSG channels were only applied for the first night.

Question

What is your diagnosis: sleepwalking or epileptic seizures?

Results of studies

Four typical events were captured on video-EEG overnight. Half an hour after falling asleep the patient sat up in bed, looked around for a few minutes and then laid back down. She did the same thing several minutes later. An hour into her sleep, she got out of bed and walked away from the camera. She was redirected by the nurse to go back to bed. Fifteen minutes later, she got up and sat on the edge of the bed for 5 minutes and then stood up, but before she could go off-camera, she was redirected by the nurse back to bed. She lay back down and for the rest of the night had no more events. She woke up twice and asked to go to the bathroom and it took 30 minutes the first time and an hour the second time to fall back asleep.

The EEG showed no epileptiform abnormalities interictally or during the events. In fact, during the events, the EEG had characteristic features of N2 sleep with abundant spindles and K complexes. She had no obstructive sleep apnea disorder (OSA) with an apnea–hypopnea index (AHI) of 1.5 per hour, no periodic limb movements, no ECG abnormalities and she had appropriate attenuation of muscle tone in REM sleep. Her sleep architecture was slightly abnormal. Total sleep time was only 384 minutes with a sleep efficiency of 78.3%. Stage N1 was 21%, stage N2 was 64%, stage N3 was 0% and REM sleep was 15%. Sleep latency was 3.5 minutes and relative REM sleep latency was 192 minutes.

Follow-up

The patient was referred for hypnotherapy and cognitive behavioral therapy (CBT) for her insomnia. Clonazepam was titrated down very slowly to 1 mg and then tapered off completely over 3 weeks. She continued to take eszopiclone 3 mg at bedtime together with her other medications. At the follow-up visit 3 months later, her daytime sleepiness had resolved, and she had had only two sleepwalking episodes since she was discharged from the hospital, one of them prior to starting therapy. She still sat up in bed nightly, but was no longer trying to get out of bed and wander. Her insomnia was still a problem, but she was working on it with the psychologist.

Diagnosis

Given these results, a diagnosis of sleepwalking, arousal disorder, was made. The daytime sleepiness was thought to be due to the intake of excess clonazepam.

General remarks

In ICSD-2 (AASM, 2005), sleepwalking is defined as a disorder of arousal characterized by short simple behavior or longer wandering episodes, with the completion of complex but purposeless tasks and memory impairment for the event.

Sleepwalking has been recognized since antiquity with mentions of it in the texts of Hippocrates and Aristotle. It has also inspired many an artist, most famously Shakespeare when he created Lady Macbeth.

Sleepwalking episodes occur abruptly usually, but not exclusively, out of stage N3 sleep during the first third of the major sleep period. Patients perform movements of varying complexity ranging from changes in position to getting out of bed and walking around, even performing complex tasks requiring manual dexterity. Rarely, behaviors can be potentially injurious leading to forensic medicine implications. During the event, although their eyes are often open giving the appearance of being awake, the person is either unreactive to or unaware of their environment or has minimal reactivity and awareness. Regardless, they appear indifferent to their surroundings, they are clumsy and their behavior is purposeless. Speech is slow and so is mentation, even though it may include full conversations. There is no autonomic hyperactivity such as screaming, tremor and sweating. Response to voices is either absent or inappropriate, but they may follow instructions to return to bed. They may be resistant and sometimes violent to attempts at waking them up because of partial arousal. Sleepwalkers are usually amnestic for the events in the morning, unless there is a complete awakening, although occasionally elaborate dream-like experiences have been reported.

Patients with sleepwalking disorder often have family histories of sleepwalking and other disorders of arousal, suggesting a common genetic factor. The HLA-DQB1*05 subtype has been reported with higher frequency in sleepwalkers. All of the disorders of arousal (sleepwalking, sleep terrors and confusional arousals) have common behavioral features and they often overlap significantly in clinical practice. There is a higher concordance in monozygotic as opposed to dizygotic twins.

Because of its prevalence in childhood and adolescence and the age-related, self-limiting nature of most cases, maturational factors are thought to play a role in the pathogenesis of sleepwalking. Medications (lithium, zolpidem, high doses of neuroleptic drugs and benzodiazepines) and recreational drugs may also induce sleepwalking. Sleepwalking tends to worsen during periods of psychosocial stress and with systemic viral illnesses and sleep deprivation, but there is no evidence that is directly due to psychiatric illnesses as previously thought; anxiety, panic and phobia seldom accompany sleepwalkers. These are all features that sleepwalking has in common with the other disorders of arousal: sleep terrors and confusional arousals. Sleep terrors tend to involve more emotional and autonomic hyperactivity but a less complex motor component, confusional arousals have low motor activity and low autonomic arousal, and sleepwalking has the most complex motor symptoms with low autonomic arousal.

The pathophysiology of all three disorders is a partial awakening from N2 or rarely from N3 sleep. There is a dissociation of motor and mental arousal characterized by the EEG findings of a mixed rhythmic delta slowing (or sleep spindles in rare cases) and a more awake EEG pattern and motor hyperactivity.

Up to 15% of school-aged preadolescents experience sleepwalking. Peak prevalence is at about 6 years when about a quarter of subjects experience one sleepwalking spell at least every fortnight. This is only an average, because most children experience sleepwalking in nightly clusters for several nights and then may go months without any. Although sleepwalking becomes less prevalent with the onset of puberty, about 10% of cases start after the age of 14 years. As far as adults are concerned, the prevalence is about 2–3%, but only 0.4% of them do it with a frequency of weekly or more. Most adults have a childhood or adolescent history of sleepwalking.

The features differentiating sleepwalking from the other disorders of arousal have been outlined. REM-sleep behavior disorder (RBD) tends to occur in older individuals, usually after the first third of the night, and has vivid dream recall associated with it. On PSG, there is preservation of muscle tone in REM sleep.

Complex partial seizures tend to be more stereotypical and also tend to occur during the day. A subtype called episodic nocturnal wandering may resemble agitated sleepwalking, but the EEG usually shows epileptiform abnormalities during the events and sometimes captures shorter events on video-EEG that fall on a continuum with the frontal lobe epilepsies. Dissociative disorders tend to have more complex and purposeful movements and the EEG during the event shows full wakefulness. Video-EEG and PSG with a full 16-channel EEG montage are therefore important diagnostic tools.

Eliminating the precipitating factor is the first line of treatment, especially if there is a clear-cut trigger such as other disorders like sleep apnea, sleep deprivation or use of pharmacological agents. Safeguarding the physical environment to prevent accidental injuries is also of extreme importance. In later-onset cases, once other disorders have been ruled out, CBT, stress management and hypnosis can help.

If there is a high risk of injury, then pharmacological agents are preferred because of fast results. These agents include low doses of imipramine or clomipramine, clonazepam, trazodone or selective serotonin reuptake inhibitors (SSRIs).

It is important to recognize that, in addition to the clinical implications, there are important forensic implications to sleepwalking. A comprehensive evaluation including PSG, video-EEG, psychological testing and necessary medical testing is important as it can have a major impact on the question of the patient's criminal responsibility.

Pearls and gold

Sleepwalking is defined as a disorder of arousal characterized by short simple behavior or longer wandering episodes, with the completion of complex but purposeless tasks and memory impairment for the event.

Sleepwalking episodes occur abruptly usually, but not exclusively, out of stage N3 sleep during the first third of the major sleep period.

Patients with sleepwalking disorder often have family histories of sleepwalking and other disorders of arousal, suggesting a common genetic factor.

Compared with other arousal disorders (sleep terrors and confusional arousals), sleepwalking has the most complex motor symptoms with low autonomic manifestations.

Eliminating precipitating factors is the first line of treatment for sleepwalking.

SUGGESTED READING

HISTORICAL

Broughton RJ. Sleep disorders: disorders of arousal? Enuresis, somnambulism, and nightmares occur in confusional states of arousal, not in "dreaming sleep." *Science* 1968; **159**: 1070–8.

REVIEW

Pressman MR. Factors that predispose, prime and precipitate NREM parasomnias in adults: clinical and forensic implications. *Sleep Med Rev* 2007; **11**: 5–30.

GENERAL

AASM (American Academy of Sleep Medicine). *International Classification of Sleep Disorders*, 2nd edn.: *Diagnostic and Coding Manual*. Westchester, Illinois: American Academy of Sleep Medicine, 2005.

Ohayon MM, Guilleminault C, Priest RG. Night terrors, sleepwalking, and confusional arousals in the general population: their frequency and relationship to other sleep and mental disorders. *J Clin Psychiatry* 1999; **60**: 268–76.

Plazzi G, Tinuper P, Montagna P, Provini F, Lugaresi E. Epileptic nocturnal wanderings. *Sleep* 1995; **18**: 749–56.

Sansone RA, Sansone LA. Zolpidem, somnambulism, and nocturnal eating. *Gen Hosp Psychiatry* 2008; **30**: 90–1.

Schenck CH, Pareja JA, Patterson AL, Mahowald MW. Analysis of polysomnographic events surrounding 252 slow-wave sleep arousals in thirty-eight adults with injurious sleepwalking and sleep terrors. *J Clin Neurophysiol* 1998; **15**: 159–66.

Case 18

An adult sleepwalker who was sleep deprived

Teresa Canet

Clinical history

Mr. X. was referred at the age of 29 years to the sleep disorders clinic to investigate motor activity and complex behaviors, sometimes aggressive, occurring during sleep over the last 8 months. He moved his hands, waved his arms, spoke loudly and sat up in bed. He once almost hit his wife. It was virtually impossible to wake him up during these episodes, and if this was achieved, he only partially recalled what had happened. The events always occurred during sleep, especially during the first part of the night, and had increased in frequency over the past 2 months, so that he was now experiencing at least one episode per week and possibly up to seven times in one night.

He had a history of sleepwalking in childhood but stopped exhibiting events after the age of 14 years. He denied smoking, drinking alcohol, substance abuse, taking stimulant medications or drinking caffeine-containing beverages. He had suffered no head injuries, or neurological or psychiatric diseases. The only surgical intervention had been a tonsillectomy. He was a musician. He usually slept 5–6 hours per night, but in recent months this had reduced to only 3–4 hours due to work schedules. The cardiopulmonary and neurological examinations were normal. His BMI was 25 kg/m². His father had been a sleepwalker in childhood and his brother had suffered somniloquy.

Special studies

The patient underwent polysomnography (PSG) because the episodes were frequent, violent and potentially dangerous to his wife.

Question

What is your differential diagnosis: complex partial seizures, REM-sleep behavior disorder (RBD), dissociative states or even malingering?

Case Studies in Sleep Neurology: Common and Uncommon Presentations, ed. A. Culebras. Published by Cambridge University Press. © Cambridge University Press 2010.

Follow-up

The patient came to the laboratory at night for PSG. He had had 40 hours sleep deprivation previously. He had been awake since his normal morning wake time the day before the PSG, which was carried out in the laboratory. He was instructed to go about his day as usual but was forbidden from taking any naps or stimulating substances during the 40 hours preceding the PSG.

The polygraphic recording was conducted on a 32-channel Cadwell polygraph with 14 channels recording EEG. Audio and video-EEG recordings were added (Figures 18.1 and 18.2). The sleep diary confirmed that he had been awake for 40 hours prior to the study.

Somnambulism (sleepwalking) was defined as partial awakening from NREM sleep, classically from stage N3, but could also be from stage N2.

Nocturnal behavioral manifestations were classified using the three-point scale of complexity of Joncas et al. (2002):

- Level 1: simple behaviors such as a change in body position (e.g. turning and resting on one's hands) or simple behaviors such as playing with the bed sheets.
- Level 2: complex behavior such as sitting up in bed, resting on knees or trying to get out of bed.
- Level 3: any event during which the subject left the bed.

An account was kept of each type of nocturnal behavioral episode.

The PSG recording started at 11.51 pm and stopped at 6.52 am. Total sleep time was 396 minutes (6.6 hours), total wake time was 25 minutes and wake time after sleep onset was 20 min. Sleep efficiency was 94%.

Sleep latency stages N2 and N3 were shortened. Stage N3 duration was increased (51% total sleep time) and REM duration was decreased (18%). He awakened 20 times and the number of arousals was 66. There was one awakening from stage N1 (5%), seven from stage N2 (35%), nine from stage N3 (45%) and three from REM sleep (15%).

There were two somnambulistic episodes, both complexity level 2, from stage N3. The first episode happened at 2.27 am. The patient sat up in bed and gestured with the expression of aggressive words; in the second episode, the patient moved his arms and hands for a short time. At the beginning of the first episode, the EEG decreased in amplitude and increased in frequency, showing irregular delta and theta activity (Figure 18.1). Hypersynchronous delta waves preceded the arousal in the second episode followed by irregular delta and theta activity (Figure 18.2). Apnea–hypopnea index was: 0.8; PLM index was: 4.8, with 1.3 arousals.

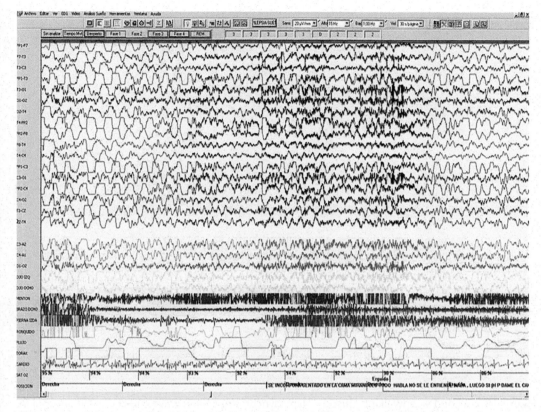

Figure 18.1 First sleepwalking episode. The EEG decreased in amplitude followed by an increase in frequency showing irregular delta and theta activity. (32-channel Cadwell polygraph. The EEG recording and electrode placement were performed according to the International 10–20 system [Fp1-T3, T3-O2, O1-O2, O2-T6, T6-Fp2, Fp1-C3, C3-O1, Fp2-C4, C4-O2, T3-Cz, Cz-T6]; 14 EEG, two electro-oculograms [EOGs], one chin EMG, one ECG, one anterior tibial EMG, one right-arm EMG, one airflow channel, one respiratory effort channel [thorax bands], one snore sensor, one oximeter and one body position. Audiovisual [including video-EEG] recording is added.)

Diagnosis

A diagnosis of sleepwalking (somnambulism) was made (classified as parasomnia: disorder of arousal from NREM sleep in ICSD-2; AASM, 2005).

General remarks

This case study describes a male adult sleepwalker with recurrence of sleepwalking events previously suffered in childhood. It is not a case of *de novo* initiation. The re-experiencing of sleepwalking after several years of remission occurs in

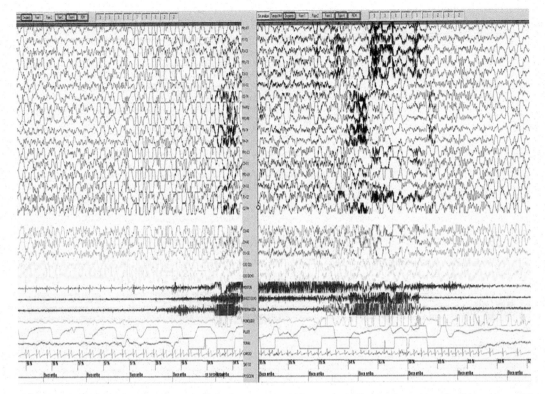

Figure 18.2 Second sleepwalking episode. Hypersynchronous delta waves preceded the arousal in the second episode, followed by irregular delta and theta activity. (32-channel Cadwell polygraph. EEG recording and electrode placement were performed according to the International 10–20 system [Fp1-T3, T3-O2, O1-O2, O2-T6, T6-Fp2, Fp1-C3, C3-O1, Fp2-C4, C4-O2, T3-Cz, Cz-T6]; 14 EEGs, two electro-oculograms [EOGs], one chin EMG, one ECG, one anterior tibial EMG, one right-arm EMG, one airflow channel, one respiratory effort channel [thorax bands], one snore sensor, one oximeter and one body position. Audiovisual [including video-EEG] recording is added.)

one-third of adult sleepwalkers. The clinical manifestations in adulthood are more complex and violent than those in childhood; this was the reason why he was referred for study.

A family history of somnambulism is highly relevant, as the prevalence in children increases to 45% if one parent is affected and to 66% if both are affected. In this case, the patient's father was a sleepwalker.

Sleep deprivation and irregular hours were the main triggers of recurrence of sleepwalking in this patient. Both factors are the most common precipitating agents. Other factors such as hyperthyroidism, migraine, history of head trauma, alcohol abuse, psychotropic medications and depressive or anxiety disorders were ruled out. Underlying psychopathology was excluded. Several recent studies have reported no clear association between psychopathology and somnambulism and have found that at least 50% of adult sleepwalkers do not suffer from it.

Diagnosis by PSG was required because the episodes were frequent, violent and potentially dangerous to his wife. Polysomnography was performed after prolonged sleep deprivation (40 hours), which increases the frequency and complexity of the motor episodes, improving the effectiveness of the recording technique and decreasing the cost of diagnosis. The most valuable findings offered by PSG were the appearance of two episodes of awakening from stage N3 sleep associated with complex body movements, which rarely occur under normal conditions in sleep laboratories. Their occurrence allowed us to establish the definitive diagnosis of sleepwalking, and excluded other diseases such as RBD, night terrors or seizure disorders, in particular frontal or temporal lobe seizures. The awakenings in stage N3 sleep are most typical, but awakenings may also occur in adults in stage N2 sleep. If PSG had been normal without motor episodes, a definitive diagnosis of sleepwalking could not have been reached.

Another result observed in this study was a delayed REM sleep latency, even more delayed than in normal people subjected to sleep deprivation. This phenomenon has been observed in the post-deprivation recovery night of sleep-walkers. This fact may be explained by the increased duration of stage N3 sleep and the increased number of awakenings in the first NREM period.

The PSG was also important to exclude the presence of concurrent sleep disorders such as sleep apnea and periodic limb movement disorder (PLMD), as both conditions can precipitate sleepwalking events by producing sleep instability secondary to arousals.

Pearls and gold

Prolonged sleep deprivation may play a role in the diagnosis of sleepwalking.
Sleep deprivation facilitates a PSG diagnosis by effectively increasing the frequency and complexity of somnambulistic events during recovery nights. This phenomenon only happens in predisposed individuals.

SUGGESTED READING

REVIEW

Joncas S, Zadra A Z, Paquet J, Montplaisir J. The value of sleep deprivation as a diagnostic tool in adult sleepwalkers. *Neurology* 2002; **58**: 936–40.

GENERAL

AASM (American Academy of Sleep Medicine). *International Classification of Sleep Disorders*, 2nd edn.: *Diagnostic and Coding Manual.* Westchester, Illinois: American Academy of Sleep Medicine, 2005.

Hughes JR. A review of sleepwalking (somnambulism): the enigma of neurophysiology and polysomnography with differential diagnosis of complex partial seizures. *Epilepsy Behav* 2007; **11**: 483–91.

Mayer G, Meissner V, Schwarzmaier P, Meier-Ewert K. Sleep deprivation in somnambulism. Effect of arousal, deep sleep and sleep stage changes. *Nervenartz* 1998; **69**: 495–501.

Pilon M, Montplaisir J, Zadra A. Precipitating factors of somnambulism. Impact of sleep deprivation and forced arousals. *Neurology* 2008; **70**: 2284–90.

Pressman MR. Factors that predispose, prime and precipitate NREM parasomnias in adults: clinical and forensic implications. *Sleep Med Rev* 2007; **11**: 5–30; discussion 31–3.

C. Other parasomnias

Case 19

Seeking food in the night

Giovanna Calandra-Buonaura, Federica Provini and
Pietro Cortelli

Clinical history

Mr. S. began having problems with his nocturnal sleep at the age of 23 when he
started to present recurrent nocturnal awakenings from sleep associated with
involuntary eating. At that time, he was attending night school and would delay
his dinner later than usual (at 11 pm). He related that he was immediately able to
fall asleep when he retired to bed; however, he woke up 30–120 minutes after
falling asleep with a compulsive desire to eat, even without feeling hungry. During
these episodes, he would wake up, rapidly go to the kitchen and then eat whatever
he found without preference for any specific food. Each episode lasted only a
few minutes and, after having eaten, Mr. S. returned to bed and fell asleep
immediately, only to wake up again several more times in the night with the same
sensation followed by the same compulsive food-seeking behavior. No accidents
occurred during the eating episodes, such as injuries in food preparation, but
sometimes Mr. S. could return to bed while eating. In the morning, he did not
always remember the eating events, but he realized he had eaten by the presence of
remnants of food. The episodes were initially rare, but in the last 15 years their
frequency had gradually increased to two to three episodes every night. He had
also progressively gained weight.

At the age of 43, Mr. S. was evaluated for his nocturnal eating behavior by an
internal medicine specialist and appropriate tests excluded metabolic, endocrine and
gastrointestinal illnesses such as diabetes mellitus, thyroid disorders, peptic ulcer and
reflux esophagitis. Mr. S. was then examined by a sleep medicine specialist. When
questioned about sleep quality, he reported sleep disruption, but rarely complained
of diurnal drowsiness and only during monotonous activities. In the evening, when
he was lying on the bed or sitting, he also reported sometimes feeling an irresistible
urge to move his legs that was partially relieved by walking. This sensation was mild
and did not usually delay his sleep onset. According to his wife, Mr. S. had recurrent
leg movements during sleep, whereas respiratory disturbances were not present.

Case Studies in Sleep Neurology: Common and Uncommon Presentations, ed. A. Culebras. Published by
Cambridge University Press. © Cambridge University Press 2010.

Mr. S. denied diurnal food intake problems, evening hyperphagia, skipping breakfast, alcohol or substance abuse, or the use of specific medication such as psychotropic or dopaminergic drugs, steroids or hypnotics, and his family history was negative for sleep or psychiatric disorders.

Examination

A general medical and neurological examination showed only a slightly increased BMI of 26 kg/m^2. Clinical psychiatric assessment excluded co-morbid psychiatric disturbances. An MRI of the head was normal.

Special studies

The sleep medicine specialist ordered actigraphic recording at home for 14 consecutive days during which the patient was required to write a subjective sleep diary, in particular noting each nocturnal eating episode. Following the actigraphic recording, the sleep medicine specialist scheduled a full-night video-polysomnogram including EEG (C3-A2, O2-A1), right and left electro-oculogram, surface EMG of the mylohyoideus muscle and a surface EMG of the bilateral biceps brachii, right triceps brachii, right extensor carpi, right flexor carpi, bilateral rectus femoris, bilateral biceps femoris, bilateral gastrocnemius and bilateral tibialis anterior muscles to investigate any pathological sleep movements. Heart rate (ECG from a standard D2 lead) and thoracic and abdominal efforts (strain gauge) were also monitored.

The sleep laboratory was equipped with a table positioned at the bedside on which the patient put the food he usually ate (bread, ham, cheese and milk).

Question

What is your diagnosis? Nocturnal manifestations of an eating behavior disorder such as bulimia nervosa? Eating behavior secondary to psychophysiological insomnia? Nocturnal eating syndrome (NES)? Sleep-related eating disorder (SRED)?

Results of studies

Actigraphic recordings for 2 weeks disclosed persistent muscular activity during the nocturnal period (between 11–12 pm and 6–7 am) and two to five episodes per night of further enhanced muscular activity (comparable to wake muscular activity) that corresponded to the eating episodes noted by the patient in his diary (Figure 19.1).

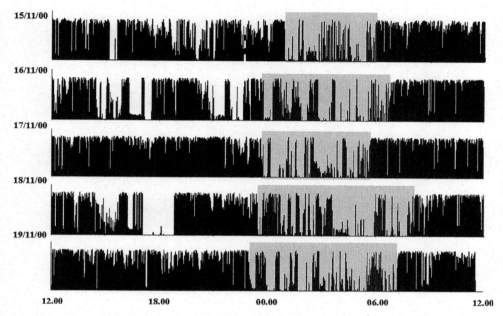

15/11/00

16/11/00

17/11/00

18/11/00

19/11/00

12.00   18.00   00.00   06.00   12.00

Figure 19.1 Actigraphic recording of five consecutive days showed an abnormal persistence of muscular activity throughout the nocturnal period (time shaded gray in the figure) and two to five episodes per night characterized by a further increase in muscle activity (of the same intensity as that presented during the day), which corresponded to the eating episodes noted by the patient in his diary.

During video-polysomnography (PSG), three eating episodes were recorded arising after an abrupt awakening from NREM sleep (stage N2 or N3) at 12.38 am, 1.43 am and 2.23 am, respectively (Figure 19.2). During the episodes, Mr. S. sat on the bed, drew the table with the food near and after a delay time ranging from 30 seconds to 2 minutes after awakening, he started to eat the food he found on the table. He ate the bread and ham and drank the milk. Food manipulation was appropriate, as was chewing during the episode. After 2–3 minutes, he fell asleep again, on one occasion with a piece of bread still in his hand (Figure 19.2). The PSG recording showed that the episode arose after awakening from sleep: EEG activity was characterized by normal alpha activity, and heart and respiratory rates were consistent with wakefulness. Mr. S. was questioned during the episodes by a sleep technician and, apart from a transient slow mentation, he was conscious during the episode. As usual, he reported feeling a compulsion to eat and specifically denied feeling hungry.

Sleep macrostructure and sleep efficiency (86%, normal value >85%) were normal. REM sleep was associated with physiological muscle atonia. Analysis of video recordings disclosed repetitive chewing and swallowing, often associated

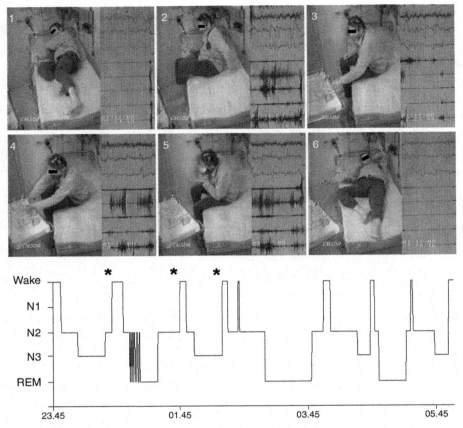

Figure 19.2 A photographic sequence of one of the three episodes recorded during video-PSG (top) and the sleep histograms of the same night (bottom). Top: video on the left and polygraphic traces on the right (electroencephalogram [02-A1], right and left electro-oculogram; surface electromyogram of mylohyoideus muscle, right biceps brachii, right triceps brachii, left biceps brachii and right extensor carpi). Mr. S. was sleeping in stage N3 sleep when he abruptly raised his head and trunk from the bed (1); after 20 seconds he sat on the bed (2), presenting some chewing movements, like a "preparatory" behavior, drew the table with the food near (3) and 2 minutes after awakening he took the bread from the table (4) and started to eat it with physiological chewing activity (5), eating for about 3 minutes. Then he lay down in bed again and fell asleep with the bread still in his right hand (6). The polygraphic recording showed an arousal from sleep followed by normal EEG alpha activity during the episode (right part of the photographs). Bottom: sleep histogram showing that sleep structure is substantially normal (N1–N3, stages 1–3 of NREM sleep) and three episodes of nocturnal eating (*) occurring during stage N2 or N3 sleep.

with EEG arousals throughout all sleep stages, but mainly during stage N2 sleep. Periodic limb movements of sleep (PLMS) were also recorded, but the PLMS index was 2 per hour (not pathological). Respiratory disorders were absent.

Diagnosis

The sleep medicine specialist established a diagnosis of SRED based on the clinical history and on the results of the video-PSG recording. The eating episodes were characterized by a compulsive desire to eat because of an "inner" feeling, without hunger, and occurred after awakening from nocturnal sleep. Moreover, there was a short latency between awakening and the eating behavior. Sleep-related eating disorder in our patient was associated with restless legs syndrome (RLS). During video-PSG, our patient did not show RLS symptoms and his PLMS index (less than 5 per hour) was normal, but during the actigraphic recording, increased motor activity of the legs during the nocturnal period was clearly evident. This was likely due to the known variability of RLS and PLMS on different nights.

Nocturnal eating disorder was excluded due to the lack of overeating between the evening meal and the nocturnal sleep onset, and the absence of sleep-onset insomnia. A daytime eating behavior disorder (bulimia and anorexia nervosa) was excluded due to the absence of inappropriate diurnal eating behaviors or compensatory strategies such as self-induced vomiting or the use of laxatives or other medication, along with a normal psychiatric evaluation.

Lastly, normal sleep latency and sleep efficiency and the brief delay between awakening and the eating behavior distinguished SRED from eating behavior in the course of insomnia, in which eating is generically performed, like other activities, in an attempt to recapture sleep.

General remarks

The specialist explained the results of the investigations to Mr. S. and prescribed pramipexole 0.18 mg of base (0.25 mg of salt) at bedtime, which can be an effective treatment to control SRED and the associated RLS. At the 1 month follow-up, Mr. S. and his wife reported an improvement in both disorders, with a disappearance of RLS and a reduced frequency of nocturnal eating episodes. The specialist increased the pramipexole dosage to 0.36 mg daily and planned a second follow-up visit after 6 months. On that occasion, Mr. S. reported a further reduction in the number of nocturnal eating episodes (only one episode per week).

Abnormal eating behavior during sleep has been described as either SRED or NES. Despite growing research, the exact boundaries between the two syndromes remain unclear. Sleep-related eating disorder is included in ICSD-2 (AASM, 2005) among the parasomnias and is characterized by recurrent episodes of involuntary compulsive eating behavior after an arousal from night-time sleep. The eating behavior is not related to hunger, but consumption of high-caloric foods or bizarre substances and bingeing is common. Consciousness is usually described as partially impaired leading to possible adverse effects (consumption of inedible or toxic substances, risks and injuries in food preparation); amnesia for the event is often reported. Sleep-related eating disorder is also associated with various medical consequences such as weight gain, obesity and dental disturbances.

The onset of SRED can be sudden and related to variable precipitating factors (traumatic life events, daytime dieting, smoking cessation, withdrawal from substance or alcohol abuse, work shifts) or gradually without any identified precipitant causes. However, the course is often chronic with a mean duration of SRED before clinical evaluation from 11 to 15 years and a frequency of at least one to two episodes nightly. Demographic data have shown a female sex predominance (66–83% of the patients in the reported series), a young age of onset (mean age 22–29 years) and a familial association.

Co-morbidity with other sleep disorders, particularly sleepwalking, obstructive sleep apnea (OSA), PLMS, RLS and narcolepsy has frequently been observed and should therefore be investigated. Psychological and psychiatric illness could also co-exist. Finally, medication-induced SRED has also been reported with psychotropic and hypnotic medications such as zolpidem in which case the disorder is fully reversed by discontinuing the drug.

The differential diagnosis should therefore include general medical and psychiatric investigations and video-PSG recordings supplemented with further channels to disclose any other sleep disorders. In SRED, the sleep structure appears substantially normal except for a decreased sleep efficiency due to frequent brief arousals. The majority of eating episodes arise from NREM sleep with a short latency between awakening and the eating behavior and are characterized by a wake polygraphic pattern. The level of consciousness during the episodes, often described as impaired, can, however, be preserved. Repetitive chewing and swallowing movements are also recorded during all sleep stages, often associated with cortical arousals and an increased PLMS index. A common pathogenic role of the dopaminergic system has been proposed to explain the association between SRED and increased motor activity, particularly in patients with RLS.

The differential diagnosis with NES, defined as a circadian rhythm disorder, is difficult as the two syndromes share several common features (nocturnal awakening to eat without control, sleep fragmentation, chronic course, familial association, co-morbidity with psychiatric disorders, weight gain and obesity). Evening hyperphagia and sleep-onset insomnia are the most useful features to differentiate NES from SRED, but misdiagnosis can still occur.

Treatment of the underlying sleep disorder, if present, is effective in controlling SRED. Low-dosage dopaminergic agents such as levodopa/carbidopa at bedtime, sometimes combined with codeine and/or clonazepam, bromocriptine and pramipexole, have been shown to reduce the eating episodes, particularly in patients with associated PLMS/RLS. Selective serotonin reuptake inhibitors (SSRIs: fluoxetine, fluvoxamine, paroxetine) have also been used with favorable effects in the treatment of both SRED and NES. Lastly, topiramate, an antiepileptic drug, has reduced night eating episodes, improved nocturnal sleep and led to weight loss in patients with SRED.

Pearls and gold

Abnormal eating behavior during sleep has been described as either SRED or NES.

SRED is characterized by recurrent episodes of involuntary compulsive eating behavior after an arousal from night-time sleep.

Co-morbidity with other sleep disorders, particularly sleepwalking, OSA, PLMS, RLS and narcolepsy has frequently been observed and should therefore be investigated.

Topiramate, an antiepileptic drug, may reduce night eating episodes, improve nocturnal sleep and lead to weight loss in patients with SRED.

SUGGESTED READING

HISTORICAL

Stunkard AJ, Grace WF, Wolff HG. The night-eating syndrome: a pattern of food intake among certain obese patients. *Am J Med* 1955; **19**: 78–86.

REVIEW

Howell MJ, Schenck CH, Crow SJ. A review of nighttime eating disorders. *Sleep Med Rev* 2009; **13**: 23–34.

GENERAL

AASM (American Academy of Sleep Medicine). *International Classification of Sleep Disorders,* 2nd edn.: *Diagnostic and Coding Manual.* Westchester, Illinois: American Academy of Sleep Medicine, 2005.

Provini F, Albani F, Vetrugno R, *et al.* A pilot double-blind placebo-controlled trial of low-dose pramipexole in sleep-related eating disorder. *Eur J Neurol* 2005; **12**: 432–6.

Provini F, Antelmi E, Vignatelli L, *et al.* Association of restless legs syndrome with nocturnal eating: a case–control study. *Mov Disord* 2009; **24**: 871–7.

Schenck CH, Hurwitz TD, Bundlie SR, Mahowald MW. Sleep-related eating disorders: polysomnographic correlates of a heterogeneous syndrome distinct from daytime eating disorders. *Sleep* 1991; **14**: 419–31.

Vetrugno R, Manconi M, Ferini-Strambi L, *et al.* Nocturnal eating: sleep-related eating disorder or night eating syndrome? A videopolysomnographic study. *Sleep* 2006; **29**: 949–54.

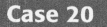
Case 20

The case of the missing loaf of bread

Cherridan Morrison Rambally

Clinical history

Mrs. P. was a 32-year-old woman who presented with sleep-related eating episodes, who had also had difficulty with sleep initiation insomnia, somnambulism, somniloquy and symptoms of restless legs syndrome (RLS) since she was 6 years old. The nocturnal eating problem was of concern to her because her weight had increased. Approximately once out of every five times she had partial recollection of the eating events. She did not eat inorganic or toxic substances, but ate loaves of bread, drank ginger ale and ate other high-caloric foods. This behavior only occurred during the night and was associated with morning lack of appetite and nausea. She denied daytime bingeing, purging, anorexia or active dieting. Somnambulism had also become of concern recently because she fell and fractured her left ankle while going downstairs towards the kitchen during one of her night-time episodes.

Typically, she had difficulty falling asleep but not staying asleep. On average, it took 1 hour for her to fall asleep, but she slept for 8 hours uninterrupted. She denied snoring or apneic episodes. She had severe daytime sleepiness, with an Epworth Sleepiness Scale score of 16 (see Appendix). If she had the time, she would take a 30–60 minute nap during the day. On weekends, she slept from 2 am to 10 am and required another 2-hour nap during the day.

Mrs. P. also complained of creepy-crawly sensations in her legs, which happened once a month and were temporarily relieved by movement. These sensations seemed to correspond to days when she was particularly fatigued. In the past, she had tried ropinirole for her restless legs with some relief.

Mrs. P. took clonazepam 2 mg BID for severe panic attacks. She had tried multiple antidepressants and antianxiety medications to no avail. Tapering down the clonazepam dose had precipitated recurrence of the panic attacks.

She was evaluated for narcolepsy in August 2004 with overnight polysomnography (PSG) and a multiple sleep latency test (MSLT). They were both normal.

Case Studies in Sleep Neurology: Common and Uncommon Presentations, ed. A. Culebras. Published by Cambridge University Press. © Cambridge University Press 2010.

The overnight diagnostic PSG showed no evidence of sleep apnea, with an apnea–hypopnea index (AHI) of 0 per hour. Mean O_2 saturation was 98%, with a nadir of 92%. There was one snore-related arousal. The MSLT showed a mean sleep latency of 11.1 minutes, with no sleep-onset REM periods.

She had a past medical history significant for Factor V Leiden, deep-vein thrombosis, pulmonary embolism, two miscarriages, gastroesophageal reflux disorder and panic attacks. She was allergic to penicillin and codeine. In addition to clonazepam 2 mg PO BID, she took aciphex 40 mg PO BID and birth control pills.

The review of systems was pertinent for fatigue, excessive daytime sleepiness (EDS), subjective weight gain, diarrhea and depression with anxiety.

Examination

Her height was 165 cm and her weight was 76.2 kg, with a BMI of 28 kg/m^2.

On physical examination, her oropharynx was moderately crowded with an oropharyngeal airway Mallampati score of class 3. The rest of the examination was normal. The patient was asleep on the examination table when the examiner entered the room, but was easily arousable and alert when engaged; otherwise, the neurological examination was normal.

Question

What is your diagnosis: sleep-related seizure disorder or sleep-related eating disorder (SRED)?

Results of studies

Overnight diagnostic PSG was performed. There was no sleep-disordered breathing with a total AHI/ respiratory disturbance index (RDI) of 1 per hour. She did have one sleep eating episode at 2.54 am, which exhibited a 30-second epoch arousal out of stage N1 sleep, followed by consuming a handful of crackers (she kept a box of crackers in bed). After the sleep eating event, she drifted promptly back into stage N1 sleep. The EEG recordings (Figure 20.1a–c) did not show epileptiform abnormalities or electrographic seizures. There was no significant sleep fragmentation, with an arousal index of 7 per hour.

Diagnosis

Based on the PSG results, a diagnosis of SRED was made.

(a)

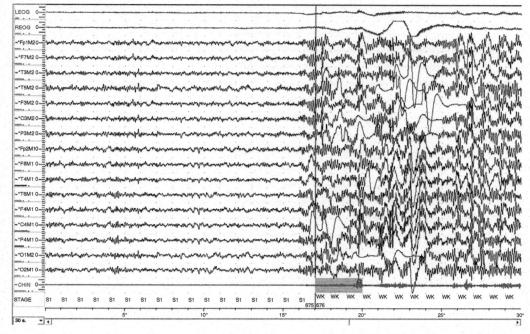

(b)

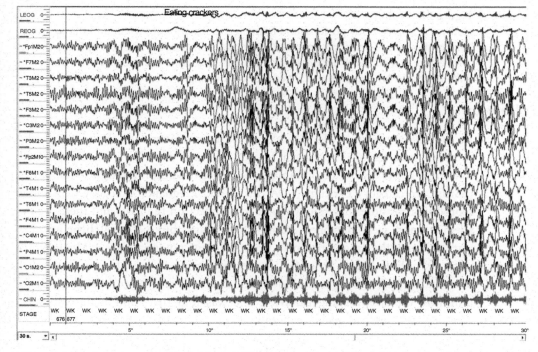

Figure 20.1 Overnight PSG with full-head EEG montage, EMG, left and right extra-oculogram and sleep stage. The respiratory parameters p flow, t flow, pulse, O$_2$ saturation, ECG,

(c)

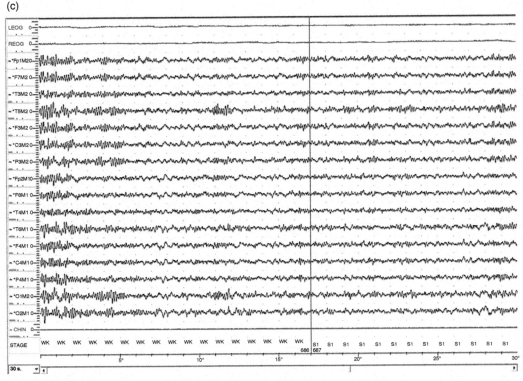

Caption for Figure 20.1(cont.)

plethysmography, body position and limb electrodes are not included in the figure. Results shown as 30-second epochs. (a) Arousal from stage N1 sleep. (b) Sleep eating is reflected as a chewing artifact in the EEG and chin EMG channels. (c) The patient drifts back into N1 sleep after 4.5 minutes of chewing.

Follow-up

At the follow-up visit, Mrs. P. informed the examiner that she was 5 weeks pregnant and taking enoxaparin for her clotting disorder. This complicated treatment of her SRED, as topiramate and selective serotonin reuptake inhibitors (SSRIs) are category C drugs (FDA definition: 'Pregnancy Category C: Animal reproduction studies have shown an adverse effect on the fetus and there are no adequate and well-controlled studies in humans, but potential benefits may warrant use of the drug in pregnant women despite potential risks.'). Medications were discontinued and, in order to prevent further injury, she was counseled to move her bed to the ground floor and leave food and water at her bedside to minimize the sleepwalking behavior. She was told that topiramate would be resumed after she had given birth and completed breast-feeding.

General remarks

Given the normal PSG and MSLT results, Mrs. P.'s EDS was most likely due to being a long sleeper with delayed phase. Her work schedule was flexible and allowed her to sleep 8.5 hours every night and to take an additional 90-minute daytime nap.

She declined treatment for the RLS, as it occurred infrequently.

Sleep-related eating disorder, also known as sleep-related binge eating disorder, nocturnal binge eating disorder and nocturnal sleep-related eating disorder, is a parasomnia that arises primarily from NREM sleep with recurrent episodes of involuntary eating and drinking. It is most common among young female adults aged 18–30. The pathophysiology is unclear, but a familial basis has been reported. Affected individuals have partial recall or total amnesia for the episodes and consume high-caloric foods or inappropriate substances. There is no daytime abnormal eating behavior such as anorexia, binge eating or purging. These episodes can lead to weight gain and obesity, if frequent. They can also lead to insomnia, excessive sleepiness from sleep fragmentation, injuries, dyspepsia and abdominal distention. Sleep-related eating disorder can be idiopathic but is usually associated with a primary sleep disorder, e.g. sleepwalking, obstructive sleep apnea (OSA), RLS, periodic limb movement disorder (PLMD) and narcolepsy. In fact, one study found SRED to be more prevalent in patients with RLS compared with controls (33% vs. 1% respectively, $p < 0.001$). Additional precipitating factors include poor sleep hygiene, variable sleep schedules, alcohol cessation, acute stress, mood disorder, substance or tobacco abuse, encephalitis, daytime dieting, travel, premenstrual state, autoimmune hepatitis and medications (e.g. anticholinergic agents, neuroleptics, lithium, triazolam and zolpidem).

The differential diagnoses include Kleine–Levin syndrome (recurrent episodes of excessive sleepiness associated with hypersexuality and increased food consumption), Klüver–Bucy syndrome (a rare disorder where individuals may place objects in their mouths and engage in inappropriate sexual behavior), hypoglycemia and nocturnal eating syndrome (which involves compulsive eating at night while awake).

According to the diagnostic criteria put forth by ICSD-2 (AASM, 2005), a patient with SRED must have the following:

1. Recurrent episodes of involuntary eating and drinking during the main sleep period.
2. One or more of the following together with the recurrent episodes of involuntary eating and drinking:
   (a) Consumption of peculiar forms or combinations of food or inedible or toxic substances. (e.g. frozen pizza, raw bacon, buttered cigarettes, cat food and salt sandwiches, coffee grounds, ammonia cleaning solutions)

    (b) Insomnia related to sleep disruption from repeated episodes of eating with a complaint of non-restorative sleep, daytime fatigue or somnolence

    (c) Sleep-related injury

    (d) Dangerous behaviors performed while in pursuit of food or while cooking food.

    (e) Morning anorexia

    (f) Adverse health consequences from recurrent binge eating of high-caloric foods.

3. The disturbance is not better explained by another sleep disorder, a medical or neurological disorder, mental disorder, medication use or substance use disorder.

On PSG, the episodes of SRED usually originate from NREM sleep, particularly stages N1 and N2, and occasionally from REM sleep. There is a short latency between awakening and the beginning of the episode (less than 30 seconds in half of the cases). There is no gross alteration in sleep structure with the exception of increased awakenings. Sleep latency may be normal or increased; REM sleep latency is normal. Sleep efficiency is decreased by 66–80%. Chewing and swallowing automatisms can be found throughout the different sleep stages, often in the form of rhythmic masticatory motor activity associated with cortical arousals. Periodic limb movements of sleep (PLMS) are typically found in patients with concomitant RLS. Most cases appear to be progressive. Complications include obesity, injuries, toxic ingestions and psychological distress with excessive weight gain. Treatment of the underlying sleep disorder, if present, is usually effective. Underlying mood disorder or alcohol or substance abuse should be addressed. Pharmacotherapy consists of administration of antidepressants (e.g. SSRIs), dopaminergic agonists or topiramate.

Pearls and gold

Sleep-related eating disorder is a parasomnia that arises primarily from NREM sleep with recurrent episodes of involuntary eating and drinking.

It is most common among young female adults aged 18–30 years.

Sleep-related eating disorder can be idiopathic, but is usually associated with a primary sleep disorder such as sleepwalking, sleep apnea, RLS, PLMD or narcolepsy.

SUGGESTED READING

REVIEW

Howell MJ, Schenck, CH, Crow, SJ. A review of nighttime eating disorders. *Sleep Med* 2009; **13**: 23–34.

GENERAL

AASM (American Academy of Sleep Medicine). *International Classification of Sleep Disorders*, 2nd edn.: *Diagnostic and Coding Manual*. Westchester, Illinois: American Academy of Sleep Medicine, 2005.

De Ocampo J, Flodvary N, Dinner DS, Golish J. Sleep-related eating disorder in fraternal twins. *Sleep Med* 2002; **3**: 525–6.

Provini F, Antelmi E, Vignatelli L, *et al*. Association of restless legs syndrome with nocturnal eating: a case–control study. *Mov Disord* 2009; **24**: 871–7.

Spaggiari MC, Granella F, Parrino L, *et al*. Nocturnal eating syndrome in adults. *Sleep* 1994; **17**: 339–44.

Striegel-Moore RH, Franko DL, Thompson D, Affenito S, Kraemer HC. Night eating: prevalence and demographic correlates. *Obesity (Silver Spring)* 2006; **14**: 139–47.

Vetrugno R, Manconi M, Ferini-Strambi L, *et al*. Nocturnal eating: sleep-related eating disorder or night eating syndrome? A videopolysomnographic study. *Sleep* 2006; **29**: 949–54.

Winkelman JW. Treatment of nocturnal eating syndrome and sleep-related eating disorder with topiramate. *Sleep Med* 2003; **4**: 243–6.

Gaining weight while asleep

Michael J. Zupancic

Clinical history

A 27-year-old woman was referred for evaluation of eating while asleep. On multiple occasions, her husband had found her in the kitchen approximately 2 hours after going to bed. She generally consumed high-caloric dessert foods during the eating episodes, but had, on occasions, eaten frozen pizza and bacon. These episodes began 3 years ago and occurred once or twice a week. She reported a 25-pound weight gain over the past several years, which she attributed to this condition. The episodes occurred more frequently during times of stress and after consumption of one to two glasses of alcohol.

She snored, gasped during sleep and awakened at least once a night with a choking sensation. She reported her sleep as "light" and felt unrefreshed upon awakening in the morning. She reported mild daytime tiredness with an Epworth Sleepiness Scale score of 11/24 (see Appendix). The symptoms had worsened over the past 3 years, which corresponded to a 25-pound weight gain. Her sleep history was significant for sleepwalking in childhood, which resolved at the age of 13.

She went to bed at 11 pm, fell asleep within 15 minutes and woke up at 6.30 am. She awakened several times a night (once to urinate) and then quickly returned to sleep. On weekends, she would sleep until 8 am. She occasionally napped for 30–60 minutes on weekends.

She had no other medical issues and denied a history of bulimia or anorexia. She had no symptoms or history of depression, anxiety or other psychiatric disease. She was not taking any medications.

Examination

She was a pleasant, overweight woman who appeared stable and not in acute distress. Her height was 157.5 cm, her weight was 79.4 kg and her BMI was 32 kg/m^2. Her neck circumference was 43 cm. Her Mallampati score was class 3 soft palate

Case Studies in Sleep Neurology: Common and Uncommon Presentations, ed. A. Culebras. Published by Cambridge University Press. © Cambridge University Press 2010.

with 1+ tonsils. Her tongue was scalloped and her hard palate was high-arched and narrow. The nasal examination was within normal limits. Cardiovascular, pulmonary, extremity and neurological examinations were within normal limits.

Special studies

The patient underwent diagnostic polysomnography (PSG).

Question

What is your diagnosis?

Results of studies

The PSG study showed the following: time in bed: 417 minutes (390–468 minutes); total sleep time (TST): 358 minutes (343–436 minutes); sleep efficiency: 86%; sleep latency: 8 minutes; REM-sleep latency: 80 minutes; wake after sleep onset: 51 minutes. Sleep stages were: 15% stage N1, 54% stage N2, 13% stages N3/N4 and 18% REM sleep. The apnea–hypopnea index (AHI) was 20 per hour and the periodic limb movement (PLM) index was 0 per hour. No abnormal behaviors were noted by video recording. The EEG showed a normal alpha rhythm on waking and no epileptiform activity was observed.

Diagnosis

A diagnosis of sleep-related eating disorder (SRED) and obstructive sleep apnea (OSA) was made.

Follow-up

The patient underwent a positive airway titration study, which showed that a continuous positive airway pressure (CPAP) setting of 8 cmH$_2$O effectively eliminated the obstructive breathing events and snoring. She was prescribed the CPAP equipment and, on a follow-up visit 4 weeks later, she reported improved sleep quality and daytime alertness. She denied eating episodes while asleep at this visit and at subsequent follow-up visits 3 and 6 months later.

General remarks

This patient suffers from SRED, which is characterized by recurrent episodes of eating after an arousal from night-time sleep with negative consequences. It is a

NREM parasomnia where one eats and drinks while sleepwalking. Patients typically consume high-caloric food in an out-of-control or "involuntary" manner. High-carbohydrate and fatty foods are preferred and bingeing is common. Subjects usually have little or no recall of the eating event upon awakening. Eating episodes can occur several times a night and do not show a circadian preference, occurring at any time during the sleep period, although they often arise during slow-wave sleep.

Preliminary data suggest that SRED is a relatively common disorder and occurs more frequently in those with daytime eating disorders. In one study, a self-administered questionnaire showed a prevalence rate of 4.6% in an unselected group of college students, 16.7% in an inpatient eating-disorder group and 8.7% in an outpatient eating-disorder group.

Most patients report consuming bread, pies, peanut butter, ice cream and chocolate and other sweets. Subjects may consume a peculiar combination of food such as butter, frozen pizzas and uncooked bacon. Reports of consuming inedible substances, such as uncooked spaghetti, egg shells, buttered cigarettes, glue and cleaning solutions have occurred in patients with SRED.

Adverse consequences of SRED include morning anorexia with abdominal distention. Weight gain, which can aggravate a plethora of other medical conditions (including OSA and diabetes), is a common consequence. Patients with SRED have sustained injury during sleep when preparing food in a dangerous manner or through consuming toxic substances. Dental cavities, from lack of dental hygiene after eating, are also a possible consequence.

A well-documented history of amnestic eating episodes during the sleep period in a person with a known history of sleepwalking is critical for the diagnosis of SRED. The sleep history should also evaluate for other co-existing sleep disorders, such as OSA. Eighty percent of subjects with SRED have another primary sleep disorder; the most common is sleepwalking. Restless legs syndrome (RLS), periodic limb movement disorder (PLMD), OSA, sleep deprivation and circadian rhythm disorders have also been associated with SRED and can aggravate this condition. As in all NREM parasomnias, alcohol can exacerbate SRED.

Physical examination should include the BMI. A careful airway examination paying close attention to the oropharynx and nasopharynx is important to look for evidence of sleep apnea. A low-lying soft palate is a frequent finding in those with OSA. The general examination should include cardiovascular, pulmonary and extremity examination. A neurological examination is also required. Several cases of eating while in a postictal state following nocturnal seizures have been described.

An attended polysomnogram (with seizure montage EEG and video) to evaluate for a co-existing sleep disorder is the standard of care, as treatment of the co-existing sleep disorder usually decreases or eliminates the eating episodes.

Occasionally, one may capture the eating episode during the study arising out of NREM sleep.

Treatment of SRED can be challenging. If the subject has OSA, as in our case, treatment of it often reduces or eliminates the eating episodes. A careful review of the patient's medications and the start of SRED symptoms is important, as hypnotic medications (such as triazolam and zolpidem) and certain psychotropic agents (including lithium carbonate) induce SRED.

Unlike in traditional sleepwalking, benzodiazepine treatment of SRED is usually ineffective and, paradoxically, may increase eating episodes. Several studies have suggested that topiramate or dopaminergic therapy, with levodopa, pramipexole or buproprion, administered in the late evening, are effective.

The differential diagnosis of SRED includes the medical conditions that can cause recurrent eating episodes during the main sleep period such as hypoglycemic states, peptic ulcer disease, reflux esophagitis, Kleine–Levin syndrome, Klüver–Bucy syndrome and nocturnal eating syndrome (NES).

Nocturnal eating syndrome differs from SRED in that subjects with NES eat during the nocturnal sleep time while completely awake. This chronic condition can be conceptualized as a circadian delay of eating with a normal circadian timing of sleep onset. People with NES are completely aware of their behavior, although they may be embarrassed by it. They often describe nocturnal eating as providing comfort. People with NES consume similar foods during the night as during the day, although they eat high carbohydrate foods more frequently at night. Unlike patients with SRED, patients with NES rarely consume unusual foods or inedible substances.

The most recent diagnostic criteria of NES include greater than 50% of daily energy intake consumption occurring after the last meal. Diagnostic criteria also include morning anorexia, nocturnal feeding and a duration of at least 3 months.

Nocturnal eating syndrome occurs in 1.5% of adult populations. Obese people are more likely to have NES, with one study showing a 0.4% prevalence of NES in normal-weight people, while 6% of those seeking weight-loss treatment reported symptoms of NES. There is an association between NES and mental illness, with a higher incidence of outpatient psychiatry patients (12.3% in one study) meeting the criteria for NES.

Several studies have shown improvement of NES with selective serotonin reuptake inhibitor (SSRI) treatment. The mechanism of action is thought to be due to the direct serotonergic effect of SSRIs in the hypothalamus, which controls circadian rhythms and feeding behavior. Several studies have shown that sertraline (50–200 mg administered before bedtime) decreases the occurrence of symptoms and results in weight loss. One small study of four patients showed that treatment with topiramate in the late evening effectively improved symptoms. Sedating agents, such as zolpidem, are not effective and, in fact, can exacerbate night eating.

Pearls and gold

Sleep-related eating disorder is a NREM parasomnia where subjects eat without control during sleep.

Patients with SRED are amnestic of the eating episode and may consume bizarre or inedible foods such as uncooked bacon or eggshells.

Sleep-related eating disorder occurs more frequently in patients with a history of sleepwalking or other primary sleep disorders such as OSA and those with daytime eating disorders (anorexia and bulimia). Treatment of the co-existing primary sleep disorder often improves or cures the SRED.

Topiramate or dopaminergic therapy with levodopa, pramipexole or buproprion, administered in the late evening, effectively improves SRED.

Nocturnal eating syndrome is a condition where patients eat during the sleep period, partly to comfort themselves while in a fully alert state. The symptoms of NES may improve with SSRI therapy.

SUGGESTED READING

REVIEW

Howell MJ, Schenck CH, Crow SJ. A review of nighttime eating disorders. *Sleep Med Rev* 2009; 13: 23–34.

GENERAL

AASM (American Academy of Sleep Medicine). Sleep related eating disorder. In: *International Classification of Sleep Disorder*, 2nd edn.: *Diagnostic and Coding Manual*. Westchester, Illinois: American Academy of Sleep Medicine, 2005.

Guilleminault C, Zupancic M. Obstructive sleep apnea syndrome. In: S. Chokroverty, ed. *Sleep Disorders Medicine: Basic Science, Technical Considerations, and Clinical Aspects*, 3rd edn. Saunders Elsevier, 2009; 319–39.

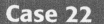
Case 22

Vivid images in the bedroom

Michael H. Silber

Clinical history and examination

A 24-year-old woman presented with a 5-year history of hallucinations during the night, occurring three to four times a week. On waking abruptly between 1 and 3 am, she would see vivid images in her bedroom, including brightly colored birds perched on her furniture, women who appeared taller than expected and a distorted man with half his head missing. The images were silent and remained still. She did not experience preceding dreams and had no idea why she had wakened. The hallucinations were realistic to the extent that she would initially jump out of bed, bruising her legs on a few occasions. Later, she became aware that the images were not real and she could remain in bed with less anxiety. The hallucinations would persist until she switched on her night light. She had not experienced hallucinations during the day and denied any delusional thinking.

She did not have a history of sleepwalking. She had not been observed to snore and no apneas had been noticed. She had not experienced cataplexy, sleep paralysis or restless legs. According to her bed partner, she did not talk, flail her arms or kick her legs in bed. She went to bed at 11 pm, initiated sleep without difficulty and woke at 6.45 am, feeling alert. She described feelings of anxiety, but had not experienced panic attacks or symptoms of depression. She had no significant past medical history and specifically did not have a seizure disorder or risk factors for epilepsy. She was not taking any medication except for a multivitamin. She worked in human resources and did not use alcohol or nicotine products. She drank one caffeinated beverage daily. She denied current psychosocial stressors and had no family history of psychiatric disorders. Her mother sleepwalked as a child. Medical, neurological and mental state examinations were normal.

Case Studies in Sleep Neurology: Common and Uncommon Presentations, ed. A. Culebras. Published by Cambridge University Press. © Cambridge University Press 2010.

Special studies

Polysomnography (PSG) was performed with an additional 16-channel EEG derivations and time-synchronized video recording.

Question

Is she having seizures?

Results of studies

The PSG study revealed a sleep latency of 11 minutes and a REM sleep latency of 99 minutes. Sleep efficiency was 81% with normal distribution of sleep stages. Her apnea–hypopnea index (AHI) was 3 per hour and periodic limb movement (PLM) index was 4 per hour. Muscle tone was normal during REM sleep. The patient awoke from stage N2 sleep at 2.05 am without any obvious precipitating cause. She described seeing a woman standing by her bed. The EEG showed an alpha rhythm commencing immediately on waking and persisting for several minutes. No epileptiform activity was noted during the event and a review of the EEG recorded over the rest of the night showed no potentially epileptogenic activity.

Diagnosis

The diagnosis was complex nocturnal visual hallucinations.

General remarks

Complex nocturnal visual hallucinations occur on waking during the night. They consist of vivid, detailed, but often distorted images of people or animals that usually remain still and silent. Fewer than 20% of patients report preceding dreams. The images persist for up to 5 minutes, but resolve if the lights in the bedroom are switched on. Patients initially believe the hallucinations to be real and may jump out of bed to confront them. However, with time, their hallucinatory nature becomes more evident and the associated anxiety lessens. A few reported PSG studies have shown that the hallucinations arise from stage N2 or early slow-wave sleep without epileptiform discharges. The events occur in association with a posterior alpha rhythm on the EEG. The frequency of events averages about twice a week, but can occur as frequently as several times a night. A few patients will report unrelated nocturnal auditory hallucinations, such as bath-running noises. Sleepwalking, sleeptalking and sleep paralysis may also be reported by some patients. The disorder is more common in women (11 out of 12 in one series).

The clinical picture of complex nocturnal hallucinations appears to be a final common pathway for a number of etiologies. In many patients, the disorder may be an idiopathic parasomnia of long duration, sometimes associated with an anxiety disorder. The hallucinations can occur in patients with narcolepsy or idiopathic hypersomnia. They can generally be differentiated from hypnagogic or hypnopompic hallucinations, which usually occur in a twilight state between wakefulness and sleep rather than in full wakefulness after sudden arousal. Images are generally less distinct than those seen in complex nocturnal hallucinations and are more often multimodal with auditory, tactile, kinetic and autoscopic components. Complex nocturnal hallucinations can result from medications, including dopaminergic agents and lipophilic beta-adrenergic agonists, and resolve if the agent is discontinued.

Certain neurological and ophthalmic conditions can cause complex nocturnal hallucinations. In Charles Bonnet syndrome, hallucinations occur with severe bilateral vision loss of any cause or at any site along the visual pathways, but most commonly with macular degeneration. Approximately 10% of patients with severe visual impairment may develop the condition. Hallucinations occur most commonly in the evening or at night, most often arising in situations with low ambient lighting. Complex hallucinations are also characteristic of dementia with Lewy bodies and Parkinson's disease-associated dementia. While they can be related to the use of dopaminergic agents, they may also appear spontaneously and can occasionally be the presenting feature of the disorder. They can occur in the day, often in conditions of dim light, or in the form of complex nocturnal visual hallucinations. Clinical clues to the diagnosis include signs of Parkinsonism, attentional or constructional deficits initially disproportionate to memory loss, fluctuating levels of awareness, depression or delusions, neuroleptic sensitivity and, in men, the presence of REM-sleep behavior disorder (RBD). Peduncular hallucinosis refers to hallucinations caused by structural lesions in the pons, midbrain or thalamus. The etiology of this disorder is commonly vascular, with hallucinations commencing a few days after a brainstem or thalamic infarct, resolving a few weeks later. Similar to Charles Bonnet syndrome, these hallucinations tend to occur most frequently in the evening. The differential diagnosis of complex nocturnal visual hallucinations includes partial seizures arising from the visual association areas. A seizure disorder can usually be distinguished from a parasomnia by the duration of the hallucinations (most seizures last 2 minutes or less), the stereotyped content of the images, associated disturbance of consciousness or automatisms, and the co-occurrence of other seizure types.

The pathophysiology of complex nocturnal visual hallucinations is uncertain. The most accepted hypothesis is that they are release hallucinations generated by spontaneously discharging neurons in the visual cortex under conditions of reduced sensory input. These conditions could include reduced environmental light, thalamic gating during sleep, or thalamic or diencephalic pathology. An alternative hypothesis is that of sleep-state dissociation, with fragmentation of the boundaries between sleep states and waking resulting in intrusion of dream-like phenomena of REM sleep into wakefulness.

Reassurance is often sufficient for patients with idiopathic complex nocturnal visual hallucinations, once it is understood that the events are benign and unassociated with significant psychiatric disease. Benzodiazepines, tricyclic anti-depressants and hypnosis do not appear to be helpful. In dementia with Lewy bodies, hallucinations are managed with reassurance, good sleep hygiene and a low level of ambient light in the bedroom. Dosage of dopaminergic medications should be reduced when appropriate. Cholinesterase inhibitors and atypical antipsychotics can be considered if the hallucinations are associated with confusion, but the potential benefits of antipsychotic agents should be balanced against their risks.

Pearls and gold

Complex nocturnal visual hallucinations occur on waking in the dark during the night.

They resolve if the lights in the bedroom are switched on.

The clinical picture of complex nocturnal hallucinations appears to be a final common pathway for a number of etiologies including medications, bilateral vision loss, dementia with Lewy bodies, Parkinson's disease and idiopathic.

Reassurance is often sufficient for management of idiopathic complex nocturnal visual hallucinations.

SUGGESTED READING

REVIEWS

Manford M, Andermann F. Complex visual hallucinations. Clinical and neurobiological insights. *Brain Res* 1998; **121**: 1819–40.

Silber MH, Hansen MR, Girish M. Complex nocturnal visual hallucinations. *Sleep Med* 2005; **6**: 363–6.

GENERAL

Fenelon G, Mahieux F, Huon R, Ziegler M. Hallucinations in Parkinson's disease: prevalence, phenomenology and risk factors. *Brain* 2000; **123**: 733–45.

Kavey NB, Whyte J. Somnambulism associated with hallucinations. *Psychosomatics* 1993; **34**: 86–90.

Teunisse R, Cruysberg J, Verbeek A, *et al.* The Charles Bonnet syndrome: a large prospective study in the Netherlands. A study of the prevalence of the Charles Bonnet syndrome and associated factors in 500 patients attending the University Department of Ophthalmology at Nijmegen. *Br J Psychiatry* 1995; **166**: 254–7.

Case 23

Noisy breathing during sleep

Roberto Vetrugno and Pasquale Montagna

Clinical history

A 24-year-old man presented with the chief concern of "abnormal breathing sounds" during sleep for the past 5 years. Medical consultation was requested because he felt socially embarrassed whenever he had to sleep with other people and because of the concerns of his parents and bed partners.

Noisy breathing during sleep was witnessed to occur in clusters, almost every night, and was not associated with any respiratory distress. The patient remained unaware of the nocturnal noise he made and continued to sleep unaffected. Coaxing the patient to change his sleeping posture would stop the respiratory noise, which could start again later on during the same night. Sudden awakenings with breathholding, gasping or choking were denied, and the patient did not report any dream content during the night with the nocturnal noise. Occasionally, he would feel tired the morning after and complained of unrefreshing sleep and/or daytime sleepiness. Alcohol and drug abuse, diabetes mellitus, thyroid dysfunction and other metabolic/endocrine disorders were absent. A clinical interview excluded relevant mood-psychiatric disturbances or sexual dysfunction.

The patient had a history of sleeptalking until 10 years of age and of recurrent episodes of transient inability to move the body as he was drifting off to sleep or immediately upon awakening from sleep, associated with a terrifying feeling. His family history was positive for sleep paralysis in the mother and for sleeptalking in the brother.

Examination

Physical examination and vital signs were normal with a BMI of $28\,kg/m^2$. His Epworth Sleepiness Scale score, for subjective assessment of excessive daytime somnolence, was 9 (normal value ≤ 10; see Appendix).

Case Studies in Sleep Neurology: Common and Uncommon Presentations, ed. A. Culebras. Published by Cambridge University Press. © Cambridge University Press 2010.

Special studies

Daytime fiberscopy of the upper airway with static and dynamic vocal cord evaluation and MRI of the brain and neck were all normal. Daytime respiratory function tests in the sitting position evaluated with static and dynamic spirometry (tidal volume, inspiratory reserve volume, expiratory reserve volume, vital capacity, forced vital capacity, forced expiratory volume in 1 second, forced vital capacity/forced expiratory volume in 1 second (%), maximal inspiratory pressure, maximal expiratory pressure, arterial O_2 tension, arterial CO_2 tension, arterial O_2 saturation, arterial blood pH and arterial bicarbonate) were normal.

All-night video-polysomnography (PSG) recordings included EEG (F3-A2, C3-A2 and O1-A2); right–left electro-oculography (EOG); surface EMG of mentalis, intercostalis (electrodes positioned in the third and fourth right intercostal space in the midaxillary line, 10–300 Hz band-passed), diaphragm (electrodes positioned in the sixth and seventh right intercostal space in the anterior axillary line, 10–300 Hz band-passed) and tibialis anterior; ECG; oro-nasal (thermistor), thoracic and abdominal respirograms (strain gauges placed at the level of the axilla and just superior to the iliac crest); microphone (on the antero-lateral part of the neck); oxyhemoglobin saturation (pulse oxymeter); and endoesophageal pressure (by means of an inflatable pressure probe transducer transnasally inserted into the lower third of the esophagus, i.e. an endoesophageal balloon). Data were acquired on a Grass polygraph with a paper speed of 10 mm/s (30-second epochs) and synchronized video recording. Sleep data were scored according to standard international criteria, including transient arousals (visible EEG arousal, usually alpha rhythm, lasting 3 seconds or longer and not associated with any stage/state change in the epoch scoring, with or without any body movements or respiratory event) with the relative arousal index (number of arousals per hour of sleep) and sleep-related breathing disorders (central [defined as cessation of respiratory effort], obstructive [characterized by continued inspiratory effort against an occluded upper airway] and mixed [an initial central component followed immediately by an obstructive component] apneas and hypopneas [a partial collapse of the upper airway and an attendant drop in pulmonary ventilation with a $\geq$30% reduction in airflow from baseline]). Abnormal motor activities were also scored including periodic limb movement while awake (PLMA) and during sleep (PLMS) and the relative indexes (PLMA-I: number of PLMA per hour of wakefulness; PLMS-I: number of PLMS per hour of sleep). Any abnormal respiratory events were considered relevant if persisting for a minimum of 10 seconds or occurring in association with an arousal and/or decrease in O_2 saturation by $\geq$3% and with a respiratory disturbance index (RDI, number of respiratory irregularities per hour of sleep) of $\geq$5.

Question

Is the patient suffering from sleep apnea or some other sleep breathing condition?

Results of studies

The patient entered sleep through NREM sleep stages, had recognizable NREM/REM sleep alternations and physiological muscle atonia during REM sleep, with a total sleep time of 222 minutes (35% stages N1/N2, 49% stage N3, 16% REM sleep) and an arousal index of 10; PLMA and PLMS were not recorded. Throughout relaxed wakefulness and NREM sleep, breathing was regular and quiet. Noisy breathing started 266 minutes after sleep onset. The respiratory sound was like a groan and occurred only during REM sleep (Figure 23.1). The groaning sounds lasted between 5 and 15 seconds and recurred in clusters, 16 minutes in net duration but spanning across 30 minutes, with the patient lying in any body position. The groaning sounds did not appear immediately as soon as REM sleep began, but rather after several tens of seconds, waxing and waning thereafter. The patient groaned during expiration only, with continuous or fragmented sounds. An EEG arousal associated with or without a change in posture often marked the onset and end of a groaning episode. The patient did not display any other kind of respiratory noises or disturbances such as snoring, stridor, wheezing and obstructive or central apneas. In particular, cessation/reduction of airflow with ongoing respiratory effort, paradoxical movements of the ribcage and abdomen, significant endoesophageal swings between inspiratory and expiratory efforts with declining O_2 saturation and audible noises, all typical of obstructive sleep apnea syndrome (OSAS), were not detected. No cessation in ventilatory effort and ventilation or awakening with short-breath sensation typical of central sleep apnea were observed. Mixed apneas were also absent.

During respiratory groaning, the pattern was remarkably abnormal because of a drastic slowing of the respiratory rate, from 14 to 6 breaths per minute, and a disproportionate increase in the length of expiration up to two-thirds of the respiratory cycle. Groaning was not associated with any discernible decrease in O_2

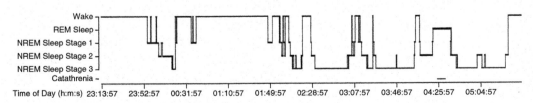

Figure 23.1 Sleep histogram showing catathrenia recurring only during REM sleep (horizontal line, bottom).

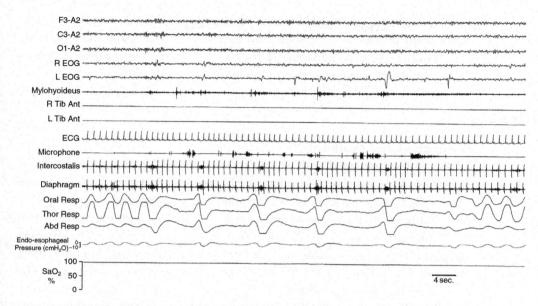

Figure 23.2 Eupneic breathing switching to catathrenic breathing during REM sleep. Note the dramatic slowing down of breathing rate during catathrenia with the cycle length now mainly occupied by the expiratory phase. Groaning sounds are shown on the microphone trace. Inspiration is associated with increased submental (mylohyoideus), intercostalis and diaphragm EMG activity, speeding of EEG frequency, waxing in heart rate and negative endoesophageal pressure. After inspiration and during groaning, endoesophageal pressure initially shows slightly positive values, thereafter returning to $0\,cmH_2O$. Diaphragm EMG activity is absent and heart rate wanes during the expiratory phase. SaO_2 remains normal throughout. EOG, electro-oculogram; Tib Ant, tibialis anterior; Oral Resp, oral respirogram; Thor Resp, thoracic respirogram; Abd Resp, abdominal respirogram; SaO_2, O_2 saturation; R, right; L, left.

saturation. During the groaning period, each inspiratory effort was accompanied by inspiratory airflow, increased EMG activity of intercostalis and diaphragmatic muscles and transient acceleration of heart rate, and by normal negative swings of endoesophageal pressure. Groaning-associated prolonged expirations were accompanied by a slight decrease in heart rate and arterial blood pressure, were not associated with intercostalis and diaphragmatic muscles EMG activity and showed an initial slight positive swing in endoesophageal pressure, the latter falling to a plateau around $0\,cmH_2O$ and remaining around $0\,cmH_2O$ throughout the groaning prior to the next inspiratory negative swing. This post-inspiratory positive raise in endoesophageal pressure during catathrenic breathing was not maintained throughout the groaning and was discernibly higher than that observed during normal expiration not associated with groaning (Figure 23.2). Episodes of sleep paralysis were not captured.

The patient was informed about his respiratory behavior during sleep, but he declined any treatment. He was clinically followed for 3 years, and still reports the occurrence of nocturnal groaning in the absence of excessive daytime sleepiness (EDS) and mood, cardiovascular and pulmonary dysfunctions.

Diagnosis

The diagnosis was catathrenia.

This patient presented with a peculiar sleep-related groaning, persistent for years. Groaning was absent in other family members, but there was a personal and family history positive for parasomnias (sleeptalking and sleep paralysis). The nocturnal groans occurred only during REM sleep, without concomitant motor phenomena and with normal arterial O_2 saturation (SaO_2). The groaning recurred every night, not associated with insomnia and dreaming, but only with a mild and not constant feeling of unrefreshing sleep and daytime sleepiness. The patient did not display psychiatric disturbances and had no signs of respiratory disease such as asthma or OSAS. He remained unaware and generally unconcerned about the problem, but he felt socially embarrassed whenever he had to sleep with other people. His parents and bed partners were disturbed and anguished by the sleep groanings.

From a polygraphic point of view, the episodes of noisy breathing were characterized by a sudden switch from an eupneic breathing to a bradypneic breathing, the latter characterized by the prevalence of the expiratory phase upon the inspiratory phase in the absence of O_2 desaturation. During this protracted expiration, a peculiar sound was produced, unlike snoring and instead consisting of a high-pitched monotonous vocal noise with quite a constant sound peak/sigh just prior to the next inspiration. This sound resembled a lament or groaning. An EEG arousal associated or not with a change of posture could mark the onset and the end of a groaning episode. It was remarkable that, during the expiratory groaning sounds, neither the diaphragm nor the intercostalis EMG were active and that endoesophageal pressure showed an initial positive rise (2–3 cmH$_2$O), subsequently returning to values around 0 cmH$_2$O. The overall clinical and polygraphic features in this patient were felt to be consistent with the diagnosis of catathrenia, a syndrome whose etiology remains unclear.

General remarks

Several mechanisms have been proposed to account for catathrenia – from central respiratory system involvement (impairment of respiratory center or persistent neonatal ventilatory pattern) to airways obstruction during expiration. There is still an ongoing debate about its nature, i.e. whether catathrenia is a sleep-related breathing disorder or a parasomnia. What this case, however, helps to emphasize is that catathrenia presents with distinctive clinical and PSG patterns and should be clearly differentiated from other respiratory disturbances with or without noise during sleep.

The respiratory tracings of catathrenia may be confused with a central apnea due to the apparent long cessation of flow and breathing effort, but careful inspection will show that, in contrast to a central apnea, where the apneic pause is preceded by an exhalation, the breath preceding the apnea in catathrenia is a large inhalation. Due to the presence of cardiac oscillations on airflow trace, the graphic may be interpreted as a "respiratory pause;" however, during catathrenia, heart rate deceleration is seen during the first part of the "respiratory pause," similar to what occurs during the Valsalva maneuver. This, together with the sound production, could be consistent with a prolonged expiration against a partially occluded upper airway. Catathrenia is also different from the physiological post-sigh apnea where a pulse artifact persists on the graphic airflow, but the gradual cardiac deceleration has its nadir during the last third of the pause.

Stridor may be expiratory too and confused with catathrenia because of its possible recurrence in clusters during the night, but stridor does not occur as a prolonged expiration following an initial deep inspiration. Catathrenia should also be differentiated from the vocalizations and moaning observed during epileptic seizures, from sleep-related laryngospasm associated with laryngomalacia and particularly from snoring. Snoring, indeed, may be also expiratory with distinctive video-PSG findings. Narrowing of the upper airway and flow limitation are not solely inspiratory phenomena, but they may occur with expiration in healthy subjects and also in snorers, in patients with upper-airway resistance syndrome and in patients with OSAS (expiratory snoring). The effect of gravity (mainly in the supine body position) on airway structures together with the relaxation of the pharyngeal dilator muscles, such as the tensor palatini and genioglossus, may promote local upper-airway narrowing during expiration more frequently at the supraglottic/retroglossal level and thus give rise to expiratory snoring. Flow limitation is associated with high frequency oscillations of the airway wall, which are propagated like a noise, i.e. expiratory snoring if during expiration. However, what clearly distinguishes catathrenia from expiratory snoring is the breathing pattern: catathrenia, unlike snoring, occurs mostly during REM sleep and displays a typical bradypneic pattern with an exaggeration of the expiratory phase. Also, O_2 desaturation does not generally occur in catathrenia and patients are not overweight. Finally, it must be noted that catathrenia remains a recently described syndrome and its full long-term prognostic implications are still obscure. Future studies should be aimed at ascertaining whether airway obstruction indeed occurs during sleep in catathrenia, as studies of the airways during sleep are still lacking.

Pearls and gold

Catathrenia occurs in expiration and mostly in REM sleep.

In contrast to central apnea, where the apneic pause is preceded by an exhalation, the breath preceding the apnea in catathrenia is a large inhalation.

Catathrenia is associated with bradypnea.

Oxygen desaturation does not generally occur in catathrenia.

SUGGESTED READING

De Roeck J, Van Hoof E. Sleep-related expiratory groaning: a case report. *Sleep Res* 1983; 12: 377.

Pevernagie DA, Boon PA, Mariman ANN, Verhaeghen DB, Pauwels RA. Vocalization during episodes of prolonged expiration: a parasomnia related to REM sleep. *Sleep Med* 2001; 2: 19–30.

Vetrugno R, Provini F, Plazzi G, *et al.* Catathrenia (nocturnal groaning): a new type of parasomnia. *Neurology* 2001; 56: 681–3.

Vetrugno R, Lugaresi E, Plazzi G, *et al.* Catathrenia (nocturnal groaning): an abnormal respiratory pattern during sleep. *Eur J Neurol* 2007; 14: 1236–43.

Vetrugno R, Lugaresi E, Ferini-Strambi L, Montagna P. Catathrenia (nocturnal groaning): what is it? *Sleep* 2008; 31: 308–9.

Sexsomnia and obstructive sleep apnea

Carlos H. Schenck and Mark W. Mahowald

Clinical history

A 32-year-old married man, accompanied by his wife, presented to a sleep physician with a chief complaint of "fondling my wife during sleep." His wife of 10 years had urged him to seek help for this problem, which had begun 4 years earlier, when he started to snore and also grope and fondle his wife sexually while fast asleep. His snoring became increasingly louder over time, and his wife commented that "he would keep trying to hump me while he was asleep." She was "shocked" to observe her husband engage in extensive sexual behaviors with her while he was fully asleep, up to four nights weekly. He never remembered these events in the morning. Non-sexual sleeptalking also appeared for the first time when he started to snore, and had persisted. His wife felt aggravated by her husband's sleepsex, which she found to be quite offensive, and it also disrupted her sleep. She doubted whether she could continue to sleep with her husband much longer and wondered whether she could remain married to him if the sleepsex persisted.

On some occasions, he would be awakened by his wife in the midst of a sexsomnia episode, and he would then recall having a sexual dream involving the two of them. His wife reported that he was somewhat insistent with his sleepsex initiatives with her, but was never aggressive or violent, and he always responded promptly to her limit setting. In general, his sexual repertoire during sleepsex mimicked the sexual repertoire during their waking lives.

Although the patient and his wife denied any underlying marital problems, the sleepsex eventually placed a major strain on their marriage. They reported having a normal sexual life and could not identify any psychosocial triggering factor for the emergence of sleepsex 4 years previously, such as sexual problems, sexual deprivation or other stress.

The patient generally fell asleep rapidly and slept (subjectively well) for about 7 hours until 6 am when he awakened to one alarm clock and got ready for

Case Studies in Sleep Neurology: Common and Uncommon Presentations, ed. A. Culebras. Published by Cambridge University Press. © Cambridge University Press 2010.

a 12-hour work shift at a printing facility. Although the patient denied any excessive daytime sleepiness (EDS), he complained of persistent daytime fatigue and tiredness.

There was no history of prior sleep disorder, and specifically no childhood or subsequent history of parasomnia, such as sleepwalking, sleep terrors, confusional arousals, sleep-related eating, sleeptalking, restless legs or rhythmic movements. There was no history of periodic hypersomnia. He also denied any family history of parasomnia or other sleep disorder. There was no history of medical, neurological or psychiatric disorder, nor any loss of consciousness or seizure-like spells. There was no history of paraphilia or criminal sexual misconduct, and he denied having problems with compulsive masturbation or excessive/inappropriate sexual fantasies or preoccupations. He denied any history of having been sexually molested during childhood or subsequently. There was no history of alcohol or substance abuse, or excessive caffeine use; he smoked a pack of cigarettes daily and lived with his wife and their daughter, but the daughter had never been involved in any of his sexsomnia episodes.

Examination

He was an alert, healthy-looking, white male in no distress. He had a normal neurological and musculoskeletal examination. The oropharynx was clear, without redundant tissue, and he had a normal neck circumference. His blood pressure was 100/58 mmHg, weight 93.5 kg, height 178 cm. A psychiatric interview was unremarkable, apart from some dysphoria over the long-standing, involuntary sleepsex with his wife.

Special studies

A hospital-based, sleep technologist-attended, "split-night" polysomnography (PSG) study was done.

Question

What should you consider?

Results of studies

The PSG study documented clinically significant obstructive sleep apnea (OSA), but no other sleep disorder or abnormal PSG finding. Sleeptalking, sleep moaning (sexual or non-sexual), sexual movements/behaviors (or any other parasomnia behaviors), rhythmic movements, periodic limb movements (PLMs), precipitous arousals from slow-wave sleep, loss of REM-sleep atonia, increased REM-sleep phasic activity, and EEG epileptiform activity were not present during either part of the split-night PSG study. The first part of the split-night study lasted 283 minutes with a sleep efficiency of 77%, sleep latency of 23 minutes, REM-sleep latency of 101 minutes, and 11.6% stage N1, 53.2% stage N2, 11.8% stage N3 and 23.4% REM sleep. The obstructive apnea index was 19 per hour, with a nadir O_2 desaturation of 78%, compared with a waking baseline O_2 saturation (SaO_2) of 97%. The average apnea duration was 22.7 seconds; the longest duration was 52.8 seconds.

The second part of the split-night PSG study lasted 183 minutes with 86% sleep efficiency. Administration of nasal continuous positive airway pressure (CPAP) at 10 cmH$_2$O pressure completely eliminated the sleep-disordered breathing noted on the baseline portion of the split-night PSG study, which resulted in normalization of sleep continuity and hemoglobin O_2 saturation. A seizure montage was employed during both parts of the PSG study with no electrical or clinical seizure activity observed. The patient was found to be pleasant and interacted appropriately with the sleep technologists throughout all aspects of his PSG study, including the 1-hour set-up time, and did not make sexual comments or act in a sexual manner.

Diagnosis

A diagnosis was made of OSA with confusional arousals and sexsomnia, together with sleeptalking.

General remarks

According to his history, the sexsomnia began in close association with the onset of snoring, and both progressed in tandem over time. As the PSG study documented clinically significant OSA, the most likely diagnosis to account for the sexsomnia is OSA inducing secondary confusional arousals with automatic sexual behavior and subsequent amnesia. In ICSD-2 (AASM, 2005), "sleep related abnormal sexual behaviors" (sexsomnia, sleepsex) is an identified variant of confusional arousals (and sleepwalking). The absence of a personal or family history of disorder of arousal in this patient, such as sleepwalking or sleep terrors, makes it less likely that he had a primary disorder of arousal responsible for the sexsomnia.

Although there was a history of dreaming associated with some episodes of sexsomnia, the preservation of the customary REM-sleep atonia during his PSG study (with a normal amount of REM sleep being recorded) virtually excluded the possibility of REM-sleep behavior disorder (RBD). This was a relevant diagnostic exclusion, as an atypical feature of this case was the reported sexual dreaming involving his wife during some of his awakenings from a sexsomnia episode. This has not previously been reported among the 31 cases in the published literature, even among the few patients diagnosed with RBD as the cause of the sexsomnia, but without any firm evidence supporting RBD as the cause of sleepsex. REM-sleep behavior disorder is characterized by dream enactment, and so it would be unusual for true sexual RBD not to have associated dreaming.

There was no history suggestive of either daytime or nocturnal seizure disorder that would raise suspicion of "epileptic sexsomnia" and the sleep EEG during his video-PSG study revealed no epileptiform abnormality and no automatisms were present. Finally, malingering was considered to be extremely unlikely.

Therefore, the final diagnoses included OSA, sleep-related abnormal sexual behaviors (variant of confusional arousals, presumably induced by OSA) and sleeptalking.

Therapy for both OSA and the presumed secondary sexsomnia was initiated with nasal CPAP at 10 cmH$_2$O pressure. At the 1-month and 3-month follow-up, the patient's wife reported that the sexsomnia had mainly disappeared since the initiation of nasal CPAP therapy, and only when the mask did not stay on his face sufficiently on a given night was he then prone to fondling or mildly groping her. The patient reported feeling less tired and fatigued during the day, and was more rested when he got out of bed in the morning. The wife was quite pleased with the response to this sleep therapy, and was optimistic about the future prospects for their marriage.

Most reported cases of sexsomnia have involved male patients with histories of NREM-sleep parasomnia (confusional arousals, sleepwalking, sleep terrors), with the sexual behaviors emerging after the parasomnias had been well established, often beginning in childhood. Forms of sexual behavior reported with sexsomnia include sexual vocalizations, masturbation, fondling another person and sexual intercourse (with or without climax). Polysomnography studies have documented NREM sleep parasomnias in these cases, although sexual behaviors have rarely been documented during PSG studies.

Seven published cases of sexual behaviors during sleep were associated with sleep-related seizures (involving sexual hyperarousal, ictal orgasm and ictal sexual automatisms) in patients with epilepsy. Therefore, abnormal sexual behaviors during sleep are almost always a manifestation of a NREM-sleep parasomnia, OSA or sleep-related seizures. Whether RBD with sexual behaviors exists is still unknown.

In the preponderance of published cases, therapy of the sexsomnia has been effective, including clonazepam for NREM parasomnias (and presumed RBD with sexual behaviors), nasal CPAP for OSA and anticonvulsant medications for sleep-related sexual seizures. Consultation with a psychiatrist or psychologist should be considered in the overall management of these cases, either to deal with personal or interpersonal/marital issues promoting or aggravating the sexsomnia, and/or to deal with any adverse personal or interpersonal consequences from the sexsomnia.

The sleepwalking variant of sexsomnia can manifest as an elaborate form of "pseudo-paraphilia" that could result in forensic and adverse psychosocial consequences.

Pearls and gold

Sleep-related abnormal sexual behaviors, with recognized synonyms in ICSD-2 consisting of "sleepsex," "sexsomnia" and "atypical sexual behavior during sleep" are a medical (sleep-related) problem, and not a primary psychological or psychiatric problem, based on the published literature.

Sexsomnia may be triggered by OSA through confusional arousals with abnormal sexual behaviors during sleep. Nasal CPAP therapy controls both OSA and the associated sexsomnia.

There is an urgent need to identify and treat these cases, as there is the ongoing potential of sexual assault on an adult or minor during sleep, with potentially tragic consequences for both the victim and the perpetrator.

SUGGESTED READING

REVIEW

Schenck CH, Arnulf I, Mahowald MW. Sleep and sex: what can go wrong? A review of the literature on sleep related disorders and abnormal sexual behaviors and experiences. *Sleep* 2007; **30**: 683–702.

GENERAL

AASM (American Academy of Sleep Medicine). *International Classification of Sleep Disorders*, 2nd edn.: *Diagnostic and Coding Manual*. Westchester, Illinois: American Academy of Sleep Medicine, 2005.

Guilleminault C, Moscovitch A, Yuen K, Poyares D. Atypical sexual behavior during sleep. *Psychosom Med* 2002; **64**: 328–36.

Rosenfeld DS, Elhajjar AJ. Sleepsex: a variant of sleepwalking. *Arch Sex Behav* 1998; **27**: 269–78.

Schenck CH, Mahowald MW. Parasomnias associated with sleep-disordered breathing and its therapy, including sexsomnia as a recently recognized parasomnia. *Somnology* 2008; **12**: 38–49.

Shapiro CM, Trajanovic N, Fedoroff JP. Sexsomnia – a new parasomnia? *Can J Psychiatry* 2003; **48**: 311–17.

Part V

Sleep-related epilepsy

The anxious hitting sleeper

Giovanna Calandra-Buonaura, Federica Provini and
Pietro Cortelli

Clinical history

Mr. A.'s sleep complaints began at the age of 15 years when he started to present
frequent episodes of sudden and unexplained arousals from nocturnal sleep
during which he abruptly raised his head from the pillow with a frightened
expression and presented violent uncoordinated movements of the limbs and
trunk. Occasionally, he would also jump out of bed. At the end of these episodes,
he usually went back to sleep. Subjectively, Mr. A. referred to being awakened by a
sensation of anxiety and tachycardia and did not remember dreaming. He was
usually unaware of his behavior, both when he awakened and the next morning.
The episodes occurred exclusively during sleep, several times per night, causing
sleep disruption and diurnal drowsiness. Over the years, the frequency of the
episodes increased from one episode nightly for 7–14 consecutive nights every
3–4 months, to several episodes many nights monthly; episodes could also occur
during daytime naps. His family history was negative for sleep motor behavior;
the patient only remembered his father talking when asleep. Mr. A. recalled being
a fearful child and later an anxious man due to a difficult relationship with his
father who suffered from a psychiatric illness. Mr. A. was born by preterm
delivery, diagnosed as a low-weight infant for gestational age and admitted after
birth for 3 months to a neonatology ward. He reported a subsequent normal
psychomotor development.

Mr. A. first described his sleep problems to his family doctor who reassured
him, explaining that these episodes were probably the manifestation of his anxiety
and no specific therapy was prescribed. However, when Mr. A. was 34 years old,
5 years after being married, the frequency, length and intensity of the episodes
increased. During some nocturnal episodes, he had unintentionally injured his
wife. For this reason, the family doctor suggested he consult a neurologist.
Emphasizing the injurious behavior during sleep, the neurologist assumed a
REM-sleep behavior disorder (RBD) and prescribed clonazepam 1 mg before

Case Studies in Sleep Neurology: Common and Uncommon Presentations, ed. A. Culebras. Published by
Cambridge University Press. © Cambridge University Press 2010.

retiring, subsequently referring the patient to a sleep medicine specialist to confirm the diagnosis. After 2 months, Mr. A. was examined by a neurologist specialized in sleep medicine. He mentioned that clonazepam had not had any effect on the frequency and intensity of nocturnal episodes. Questioned about any sleep-related respiratory disturbances, Mr. A.'s wife replied that the patient usually snored and would sometimes seem to stop breathing for a few seconds during sleep.

Examination

General medical and neurological examinations showed a mildly elevated BMI of $28 \, kg/m^2$.

Special studies

The sleep medicine specialist ordered a full-night video-polysomnography (PSG) recording including standard bipolar EEG (according to the International 10–20 system), right and left electro-oculograms (EOGs), surface EMG of the mylo-hyoideus muscle, ECG (from a standard D2 lead), oro-nasal, thoracic and abdominal respirograms, and circulating oxyhemoglobin saturation. He also suggested a 3T MRI of the head.

Question

What is your diagnosis? Nocturnal panic attacks? RBD? Obstructive sleep apnea (OSA)-induced confusional arousals? Epileptic seizures?

Follow-up

The specialist decided to withdraw clonazepam and advised Mr. A. not to drive due to his diurnal drowsiness until the results of the investigations became available and appropriate therapy was prescribed.

Results of studies

During video-PSG, 30 episodes were recorded and recognized by Mr. A.'s wife as those usually presented by the patient. Episodes were characterized by an abrupt arousal from sleep with stereotypical motor behaviors of increasing complexity. During the shortest episodes, the patient raised his head and sometimes his shoulders from the bed with his eyes open and then fell asleep again. During the complex ones, Mr. A. raised his head and trunk and then grasped the bed with

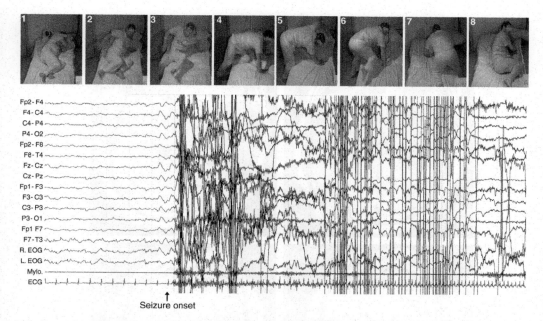

↑
Seizure onset

Figure 25.1 A photographic sequence of a typical episode of Mr. A. (top) and the corresponding polygraphic recordings (bottom) during video-PSG. Mr A. is sleeping in stage N2 sleep (1) (see PSG traces at the bottom of the figure). He abruptly raises his head and trunk from the bed (2), jumps out of bed (3), turns his body to the right and puts his knee on the bed (4). He moves his left arm violently, drawing a circle (5), then turns his body to the right again, climbing onto the bed (6) and then getting off the other side of the bed (7). At the end of the seizure, Mr. A. gets back into bed (8). The PSG recordings show that episode onset coincides with the appearance of a K-complex; EEG tracings are then masked by muscular artifacts. Tachycardia appears synchronously with movement onset. EEG (Fp2-F4, F4-C4, C4-P4, P4-O2, Fp2-F8, F8-T4, Fz-Cz, Cz-Pz, Fp1-F3, F3-C3, C3-P3, P3-O1, Fp1-F7, F7-T3); R., right; L., left; EOG, electro-oculogram; Mylo., mylohyoideus muscle; ECG, electrocardiogram (from a standard D2 lead). Paper speed: 30 mm/s.

one hand, turned his body alternately to one side or the other, moved his pelvis in an anterior–posterior direction and presented repetitive movements with his arms and legs. He could also sit on the bed; on one occasion, he jumped out of bed (Figure 25.1). Episodes occurred in all NREM-sleep phases (mainly in phase 2) and lasted from 2 to 30 seconds.

EEG ictal recordings did not disclose any epileptic abnormalities before or during the episodes. Motor behavior coincided with the appearance of a K-complex and soon EEG tracing was masked by muscular artifacts. Autonomic changes (tachycardia and irregular respiration) coincided with movement onset. Interictal EEG was normal.

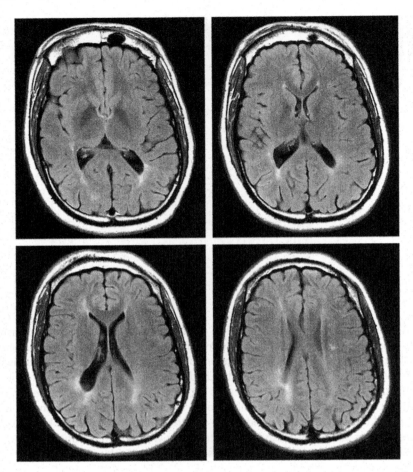

Figure 25.2 Axial FLAIR (fluid-attenuated inversion recovery) T2-weighted images of the brain showed bilateral hyperintense periventricular lesions and asymmetrical enlargement of the occipital ventricles due to perinatal damage.

A reduction in nocturnal sleep efficiency (66%; normal value, >85%) due to frequent arousals and a prevalence of light sleep were documented; REM-sleep latency was increased (180 minutes). REM sleep was associated with physiological muscle atonia. Snoring and OSAs were also observed in all sleep phases with an apnea–hypopnea index (AHI) of 23 per hour (nadir oxyhemoglobin saturation, 79%; mean apnea–hypopnea duration, 29 seconds). The onset of the motor episodes was sometimes preceded by an episode of apnea, but in the majority of cases, the motor behavior was independent of the respiratory disturbance.

A brain MRI showed hyperintensity of the frontal and occipital periventricular white matter on T2-weighted images, suggestive of leukoencephalopathy, probably due to perinatal damage (Figure 25.2).

Diagnosis

The sleep medicine specialist established a diagnosis of nocturnal frontal lobe epilepsy (NFLE) based on historical features (onset of episodes in adolescence, increased frequency of the episodes with age, occurrence of many episodes per night, every night) and video-PSG findings (episodes characterized by brief duration, and stereotyped and violent motor behavior; episodes of different complexity, but with the same motor onset; episode onset mainly during stage N2 sleep).

Nocturnal panic attacks are described as abrupt awakenings associated with rapid alertness and behavioral manifestations of great fear (shortness of breath, tachycardia, palpitations, chest discomfort). They usually last several minutes with a progressive increase in fear, often associated with identical manifestations during wakefulness and not associated with stereotypical violent motor behaviors as with the episodes documented during Mr. A.'s video-PSG. Documentation of the physiological muscular atonia during REM sleep with video-PSG and the absence of dream mentation associated with the episodes excluded the diagnosis of RBD. Finally, Mr. A. had mild OSA disorder. Obstructive sleep apnea was not the cause of the episodes recorded during Mr. A.'s video-PSG, as most events did not follow an apnea. However, the respiratory disorder causing sleep instability due to frequent arousals could be a trigger for seizure occurrence.

General remarks

At the follow-up visit, the specialist explained to Mr. A. the results of the investigations and the features and prognosis of NFLE, and prescribed carbamazepine 400 mg at bedtime. He also explained that Italian law prohibits driving until patients have been seizure-free for 2 years (6 months in New York State). Moreover, he recommended that Mr. A. lose weight to improve his sleep-related respiratory disorder, given his refusal to use CPAP.

At the second follow-up visit, Mr. A. and his wife reported a marked reduction in the frequency of the nocturnal episodes with carbamazepine (only one episode in 3 months) and disappearance of the excessive daytime sleepiness (EDS). The specialist scheduled a third follow-up visit and a carbamazepine blood level evaluation after 6 months, and explained to Mr. A. that an increase in drug dosage would have been necessary in case of seizure reappearance.

Nocturnal frontal lobe epilepsy is a peculiar partial epilepsy whose clinical features comprise a spectrum of paroxysmal motor manifestations of variable duration and complexity, occurring mainly during sleep. Three main semiological patterns were observed in a large series studied by video-PSG recordings: (1) minor motor events characterized by brief, sudden and recurrent arousals from sleep associated with a frightened or surprised expression and stereotyped movements of the head, trunk and limbs (paroxysmal arousals); (2) major attacks, originally named nocturnal paroxysmal dystonia, that include asymmetric bilateral tonic seizures and more complex motor episodes with violent, uncoordinated and repetitive movements of the limbs and trunk and vocalizations; and (3) more prolonged episodes with epileptic nocturnal wandering, consisting of a stereotypic paroxysmal ambulatory behavior. These three different manifestations may co-exist in the same patient and are thought to reflect different duration, amplitude and spread of the epileptic discharge. The beginning of the ictal motor manifestation is usually stereotyped in the same patient.

Seizures can occur during any time of the night, mainly from NREM sleep stages N1 and N2. Interictal or ictal EEG findings are often normal or non-specific in NFLE patients leading to problems of differential diagnosis between epileptic and non-epileptic paroxysmal sleep-related behaviors. Video-PSG together with careful history taking is necessary to establish a correct diagnosis.

Nocturnal frontal lobe epilepsy can occur sporadically or as an inherited form associated with mutations in the genes encoding the α4 (CHRNA4), β2 (CHRNB2) and α2 (CHRNA2) subunits of the neuronal nicotinic acetylcholine receptors (autosomal dominant NFLE, or ADNFLE). Clinically, sporadic and familiar cases of NFLE have a similar presentation. A positive family history for one or more parasomnias is common in patients with NFLE.

Seizure frequency in NFLE is usually high (almost every night, several times per night). Patients are not always aware of their nocturnal attacks, but they often report sleep discontinuity and EDS. Prognosis of the disease is partially benign, as most patients respond favorably to antiepileptic drugs. Carbamazepine is the drug of choice and is effective at low doses in most patients, but fails to modify seizure frequency in about 30% of cases. In addition to carbamazepine, patients may respond to topiramate. Patients with drug-resistant disabling seizures should be considered for resective surgery of the epileptogenic zone that may effectively control seizures and epilepsy-related sleep disturbances. An accurate presurgical evaluation with deep implanted electrodes is required to identify the epileptogenic zone.

Pearls and gold

Nocturnal frontal lobe epilepsy is a peculiar partial epilepsy with a clinical spectrum of paroxysmal motor manifestations of variable duration and complexity, occurring during sleep.

Manifestations include brief, sudden and recurrent arousals from sleep associated with a frightened or surprised expression and stereotyped movements of the head, trunk and limbs (paroxysmal arousals); asymmetric bilateral tonic seizures and complex motor episodes with violent repetitive movements of the limbs and vocalizations (originally called nocturnal paroxysmal dystonia); and stereotypic paroxysmal ambulatory behavior (epileptic nocturnal wandering).

Seizures can occur at any time of the night, mainly from NREM sleep stage N2.

Conventional EEG ictal or interictal recordings generally fail to show epileptiform activity.

SUGGESTED READING

HISTORICAL

Lugaresi E, Cirignotta F. Hypnogenic paroxysmal dystonia; epileptic seizures or a new syndrome? *Sleep* 1981; **4**: 129–38.

REVIEW

Tinuper P, Provini F, Bisulli F, *et al.* Movement disorders in sleep: guidelines for differentiating epileptic from non-epileptic motor phenomena arising from sleep. *Sleep Med Rev* 2007; **11**: 255–67.

GENERAL

Nobili L, Francione S, Mai R, *et al.* Surgical treatment of drug-resistant nocturnal frontal lobe epilepsy. *Brain* 2007; **130**: 561–73.

Oldani A, Manconi M, Zucconi M, Martinelli C, Ferini-Strambi L. Topiramate treatment for nocturnal frontal lobe epilepsy. *Seizure* 2006; **15**: 649–52.

Provini F, Plazzi G, Tinuper P, *et al.* Nocturnal frontal lobe epilepsy. A clinical and polygraphic overview of 100 consecutive cases. *Brain* 1999; **122**: 1017–31.

Scheffer IE, Bhatia KP, Lopes-Cendes I, *et al.* Autosomal dominant nocturnal frontal lobe epilepsy: a distinctive clinical disorder. *Brain* 1995; **118**: 61–73.

Bad dreams

Philip King

Clinical history

A 54-year-old man reported that he had been having problems with his sleep for
the previous 20 years. He said he had "bad dreams." These consisted of seeing a
dark hole in the ground as if dug for a pit or grave. The size and position of the
hole with respect to him changed, but only slightly from episode to episode. He
always had a feeling that he was about to fall into the hole. Sometimes during
these episodes he would lash out with his upper or lower limbs and his wife, who
was sleeping with him, was often struck. She was never part of the dreams and she
told him that the activity was never specifically directed towards her. The episodes
were almost all in bed, but occasionally he found himself on the floor beside the
bed. He had never found himself in other areas of the house or bedroom. He had
partial awareness of limb and body movements during the episodes that he could
not control. He thought they lasted a minute or two. He did not remember
vocalization or talking during the episodes. He thought he usually had about one
episode per night, but he was occasionally aware of having up to three. They
typically occurred about 30 minutes after sleep onset or around 4–5 am. There
was never tongue biting or incontinence.

He had noted mild sleepiness during the day since his teens. In the years
following the onset of the night episodes, his daytime sleepiness became worse.
He snored and was overweight. About 8 years before presentation, he underwent
a sleep study and was told he had sleep apnea that was "not obstructive." He
subsequently commenced fixed pressure nasal continuous positive airway pressure (CPAP), but used it only intermittently. He did not think it had a significant
impact on the frequency or nature of the night episodes, and his daytime
sleepiness did not improve.

He started having episodes during the day about 15 years prior to presentation
consisting of an unusual feeling in the head and speech arrest if he was talking at
the onset. He did not think he lost awareness during these episodes. He took

Case Studies in Sleep Neurology: Common and Uncommon Presentations, ed. A. Culebras. Published by
Cambridge University Press. © Cambridge University Press 2010.

carbamazepine and the day episodes stopped and did not recur, despite later ceasing taking the drug. Carbamazepine had no impact on the night episodes, but he subsequently started having visual hallucinations of seeing a child or cat in the bed beside him when it was dark. These symptoms persisted when the carbamazepine was ceased.

Eight months prior to presentation he commenced gabapentin, started losing weight and, without physician advice, obtained and started using an adaptive servo-ventilator device (VPAP Adapt SV). He reported an improvement in the night episodes, but they still occurred on several nights per week. The visual hallucinations ceased.

He had a detailed knowledge of engineering and computer programming. He did not smoke or use alcohol and he denied use of recreational drugs. His only medication apart from gabapentin was an ACE inhibitor (ramipril) for hypertension. There was no history of cardiac or respiratory disease.

Examination

On examination, the patient was obese. His height was 177 cm and weight 113 kg, yielding a BMI of 36 kg/m². The oral airway was small and reddened. A detailed neurological examination was completely normal. Cardiac and respiratory examinations were also normal.

Special studies

An MRI scan and EEG were carried out. Overnight video-polysomnography (PSG) was planned. The patient was very reluctant to consider changing the servo-ventilator device he had purchased from his own funds, so it was decided to perform the study using his machine.

Question

What is your diagnosis: seizure or parasomnia?

Results of studies

The MRI of the brain was normal. The EEG showed occasional 1-second or so runs of moderate amplitude (2–5 Hz) slowing in either temporo-frontal region during early drowsiness. Also, during drowsiness, several approximately 2-second bursts of moderate amplitude 3 Hz anterior predominant slowing were seen.

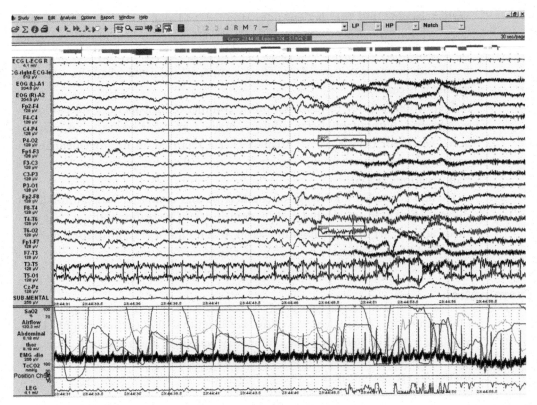

Figure 26.1 Seizure onset in the patient from stage N2 sleep showing return of alpha waves and the onset of symmetrical centrofrontal fast activity, which was thought to be EMG and/or normal beta activity. There were no specific features (focal onset, recruitment) to suggest a seizure. Note the tachycardia. An artifact is present from the left posterior temporal electrode (T5) throughout. Vertical lines indicate 0.5 seconds of recording time (30 seconds displayed).

During the video-PSG, the patient had four almost identical events. These consisted of sudden stiffening of the upper limbs with the elbows extended. In the first, the upper limbs were raised above the head, but in the others they were close to the body although it was noted in these that he was gripping the rails beside the bed. No vocalization was noted. The episodes lasted 5 seconds. The PSG showed stage N2 sleep before all the events and was identical in each. The event started with the return of posterior predominant alpha waves and the onset of symmetrical centrofrontal fast activity, which was thought to be EMG and/or normal beta activity. There were no specific features (focal onset, recruitment) to suggest a seizure. Tachycardia was noted. There was no postictal slowing (Figure 26.1). Sleep onset was at 11.12 pm. The first event occurred 14 minutes after sleep onset at 11.26 pm and subsequent events occurred at 11.44 pm, 3.15 am and 5.38 am. All stages of sleep were recorded. No significant apneas or O_2 desaturation were seen with the use of the patient's own machine.

The patient obtained a home video of an event. This was different to the events recorded in the sleep laboratory. The onset was similar and consisted of sudden stiffening of the upper limbs with the elbows extended. On this occasion, the shoulders were abducted to about 90°. Subsequently, some clonic movements were noted, superimposed on the predominant tonic posture of the upper limbs. After about 1 minute, the extended upper limbs moved in a semi-rhythmic circular fashion interrupted by clonic movements and repetitive arching of the back, and thrusting movements of the lower limbs were seen. The episode occurred about 1 hour after the patient lay down to sleep and lasted 1.5 minutes. Vocalization was noted during the episode. The patient seemed immediately responsive after the episode and got out of bed and turned off the video.

Follow-up

The episodes were thought to be frontal lobe seizures leading to a diagnosis of nocturnal frontal lobe epilepsy (NFLE). No specific diagnosis was reached concerning the other visual hallucinations. Breathing was not significantly impaired at night using the patient's servo-ventilator device and so the underlying breathing disorder, if present, was unknown. Obstructive sleep apnea (OSA) was felt very likely. The previously diagnosed apnea that was "not obstructive" was likely to be central sleep apnea associated with the undiagnosed seizures.

The patient did not wish to take carbamazepine again. Levetiracetam was commenced and the dose incremented. The patient reported a marked reduction in the frequency of events down to one episode per week with a dose of 500 mg in the morning and 1000 mg at night. Unfortunately, during one episode he fell out of bed again and on this occasion he injured his shoulder. Plans were made to increase the evening dose further and, if events were controlled, to taper and cease the gabapentin.

Diagnosis

The diagnosis was NFLE with central sleep apnea (due to seizures).

General remarks

The differential diagnosis of these nocturnal events includes NREM-sleep-arousal parasomnias, REM-sleep behavior disorder (RBD) and psychogenic disorders.

NREM-sleep-arousal parasomnias are the disorders that most closely mimic NFLE and cause diagnostic difficulty. They include confusional arousals, sleep terrors and sleepwalking. Various elements of these named disorders may be seen in any single NREM-sleep-arousal parasomnia episode and so they are best regarded as a continuum of disorders. The episodes are not highly stereotyped. What the sufferer does during the episodes varies from event to event, most notably with sleepwalking. The events typically occur 1 hour after sleep onset during the first slow-wave sleep period. They may occur later in the night, but would not be expected within the first 30 minutes of sleep. The frequency varies, but several events per month is typical for those who come to close medical attention. By contrast, the average frequency of events in patients with NFLE is 20 per month, and in patients having nightly episodes, the mean number of episodes per night was three (Provini *et al.*, 1999). Other points in favor of a diagnosis of NFLE compared with parasomnia in the patient include short duration and recall of episodes.

REM-sleep behavior disorder events consist of violent motor activity and vocalization (talking, shouting and often swearing), accompanied by a dream where the activity is appropriate to the content of the dream. The dream usually has a violent content and the theme usually varies from episode to episode. This is most unlike this patient where the content of his "bad dream" was highly stereotyped. By definition, RBD occurs exclusively in REM sleep, and the events occur most frequently later in the sleep period when REM sleep is more common; the earliest would be after the first hour of sleep during the first period of REM sleep. This is also most unlike this patient, where the first recorded episode occurred 30 minutes after sleep onset. Nightly episodes and up to three episodes per night is also against a diagnosis of RBD. Injury to the RBD sufferer or bed partner does occur frequently in RBD, as was seen with this patient.

Possible psychogenic disorders would include malingering, nocturnal panic disorder or a dissociative state. These were thought unlikely because of the absence of a psychiatric history and lack of secondary gain. Indeed, the events were very disruptive to the patient's sleep and had caused injury. Nevertheless, a psychiatric cause could not be ruled out solely on the clinical information.

The clinical and video-PSG features of NFLE have been described in detail in the literature. Based on clinical features, these are classified as paroxysmal arousals, nocturnal paroxysmal dystonia and episodic or epileptic nocturnal wanderings. Using clinical information alone, a scale has been developed that appears to be accurate for differentiating NFLE from parasomnia. This may be particularly useful where video-PSG studies are not readily available.

The video-PSG and the home study were very helpful in the diagnosis of this patient. The recording of four episodes that were highly stereotyped both clinically and on EEG makes the diagnosis of seizure certain, despite the absence of ictal EEG features. Patients with NFLE may be partially responsive and able to carry out some voluntary movements during the episodes. It was felt that the gripping of the handrails was probably voluntary, preventing involuntary abduction of the shoulders as was seen in the first recorded episode. The features were those of the paroxysmal arousal subgroup of NFLE. The event recorded at home was typical of the nocturnal paroxysmal dystonia subgroup. When these occur in the same patient, the onset of the seizure is similar for both types. The ictal EEG is often obscured by movement and muscle artifacts, but otherwise frequently shows features of an arousal without clear seizure activity. In some cases, theta or delta slowing, fast activity or focal or diffuse flattening is seen. When the changes on the EEG in the anterior head regions at the onset of the event are symmetrical, it is usually impossible to distinguish seizure from arousal activity with certainty. Focal or unilateral onset and a progressive increase in amplitude and decrease in frequency of the activity make it more likely that it is seizure activity and not just an arousal. No postictal slowing is characteristic of the seizures of NFLE. Sometimes seizures of temporal lobe origin may spread to the frontal lobe in a way that completely mimics what is seen clinically and on the EEG in NFLE. In patients with psychogenic nocturnal events, there is usually evidence of an arousal or awakening prior to the onset, but the diagnosis can be difficult in some cases.

When a diagnosis of NFLE is made, an MRI should be performed because the frontal lesion, if present, may be subtle. There should be a rigorous search of the family history, which may not be apparent on initial questioning. Some families of patients with familial NFLE have mutations of the genes responsible for encoding the A4 or B2 subunits of the acetylcholine receptor, increasing their sensitivity.

Carbamazepine is the drug of choice for NFLE, but when it is not efficacious, other drugs used for the partial epilepsies may be considered. There are no drug trials that aid choice of drug. Sleep apnea may trigger seizures in some patients and it should be diagnosed and treated appropriately.

Pearls and gold

The NREM arousal parasomnias are the disorders that most closely mimic NFLE and cause diagnostic difficulty.

The average frequency of events in patients with NFLE is 20 per month, and in patients having nightly episodes the mean number of episodes per night is three.

Based on clinical features, NFLE events are classified as paroxysmal arousals, nocturnal paroxysmal dystonia and episodic or epileptic nocturnal wanderings.

Patients with NFLE may be partially responsive and able to carry out some voluntary movements during the episodes.

Carbamazepine is the drug of choice for NFLE, but when it is not efficacious, other drugs used for the partial epilepsies may be considered.

SUGGESTED READING

REVIEW

Provini F, Plazzi G, Tinuper P, *et al.* Nocturnal frontal lobe epilepsy. A clinical and polygraphic overview of 100 consecutive cases. *Brain* 1999; **122**: 1017–31.

GENERAL

Derry CP, Davey M, Johns M, *et al.* Distinguishing sleep disorders from seizures: diagnosing bumps in the night. *Arch Neurol* 2006; **63**: 705–9.

Shouse MN, Mahowald MW. Epilepsy, sleep and sleep disorders. In: Kryger MH, Roth T, Dement WC, eds. *Principles and Practice of Sleep Medicine.* Philadelphia: Elsevier Saunders, 2005; 863–78.

Tinuper P, Provini F, Bisulli F, *et al.* Movement disorders in sleep: guidelines for differentiating epileptic from non-epileptic motor phenomena arising from sleep. *Sleep Med Rev* 2007; **11**: 255–67.

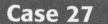

Case 27

Sleepwalking or seizing?

Mark Eric Dyken and Deborah C. Lin-Dyken

Clinical history

An 8-year-old female presented to a pediatric neurology clinic for evaluation of chronic sleep-related behaviors that were unresponsive to anticonvulsant treatment. The patient had been 8 lbs, 1 oz at birth following a forceps-assisted vaginal delivery. Developmentally, she attained normal milestones and walked at 9 months of age. Her surgical history was significant for a tonsillectomy with adenoidectomy at 6 years of age.

At 2 years of age, she began waking from naps and would "climb out of her crib and act like she couldn't breathe." During these events, the patient would move all over the bed, and was often found on the floor with whole-body "back and forth" rocking. At these times, she would remain unresponsive to commands for up to 60 seconds, after which she would "wake up" and ask why she was in a place other than her bed. Afterwards, the patient frequently spoke in a confused manner, often pointing to her pillow and repeatedly asking, "What is this?" until she was answered, after which she would respond, "Oh."

Occasionally she would awaken her parents with choking and gagging noises. At these times, she would be found in "a state of unawareness" and "wandering" to the bathroom. The frequency of these walking episodes increased during periods of stress up to two to three times a night, five nights a week, after which they might resolve "for a long time."

All events arose from sleep and none was associated with frank lateralizing signs, tonic/clonic activity, incontinence or cyanosis. The day after a spell, the patient behaved and functioned normally, but remained amnestic for all of the reported events.

An EEG at that time was normal. Nevertheless, a concern for seizure dictated a trial of phenobarbital, which resulted in behavioral problems that necessitated a change to diphenylhydantoin. This had no effect on the spells, which continued at an average frequency of once per week.

At 7 years of age, as the nocturnal behaviors continued, another EEG was performed and again was read as normal. A change in the anticonvulsant therapy

Case Studies in Sleep Neurology: Common and Uncommon Presentations, ed. A. Culebras. Published by Cambridge University Press. © Cambridge University Press 2010.

to carbamazepine had no effect on the spells. Moreover, when carbamazepine was combined with diphenylhydantoin, the sleep-related events worsened.

The patient's family history was significant for seizure disorders and parasomnias. Her father was diagnosed with a partial complex seizure disorder at the age of 12 years and was treated with diphenylhydantoin. He had been seizure free for over 6 years. Her paternal grandmother and two paternal cousins had suspected seizures that required the temporary use of anticonvulsants with spontaneous resolution. Her mother and two maternal cousins were noted to have parasomnias (sleepwalking).

Given the patient's two normal EEGs, the ineffectiveness of anticonvulsants and the family history of sleepwalking, the parents raised concerns about a parasomnia. Their worry regarding the potential untoward effects of unnecessary medication led to their weaning the patient off anticonvulsant therapy.

After initially discontinuing therapy, the patient's personality improved and she had fewer episodes of sleepwalking-like events. However, after 8 days off therapy, she had a 1-minute nocturnal episode characterized by jerking of all four extremities, followed by a 1-hour period of staring and tremulousness. To address this issue, her neurologist ordered polysomnography (PSG) with split-screen video-PSG analysis to evaluate for parasomnia or seizure.

Examination

On simple observation, the patient was a pleasant, otherwise healthy girl, aged 8 years and 10 months. Her vital signs and anthropometric data (which included a height of 128.5 cm, a weight of 30.7 kg and a head circumference of 52.5 cm) were unremarkable. Her oropharyngeal, nasal, general and neurological examinations revealed no focal abnormalities.

Special studies

A waking EEG was read as normal. Standard video-PSG captured seven of the patient's classic spells and was considered diagnostic.

Question

What is your diagnosis: somnambulism or seizure disorder?

Results of studies

The PSG study started with a lights-out time at 9.44 pm; the patient's routine bedtime was 8.30 pm. Her mother, present throughout the entire study, confirmed that the seven events captured were typical of previously reported behaviors. Only the first spell arose from stage N3 sleep. The remaining six events began in stage

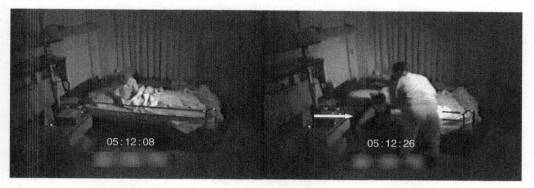

Figure 27.1 Video-EEG of a typical spell: after suddenly sitting up (left picture), the patient demonstrates stereotypical tonic posturing of the extended right upper extremity (indicated by the arrow in the picture to the right), followed by clonic activity of all four extremities. The relatively violent nature of the spells aroused the technicians' concern and encouraged their physical presence during the event. This allowed for a detailed account of every spell and a thorough clinical assessment during each postictal state.

N2 sleep. The episodes occurred at 11.08 pm (90-second duration), 11.52 pm (45-second duration), 12.29 am (90-second duration), 1.09 am (90-second duration), 4.19 am (60–90-second duration), 5.12 am (120-second duration) and 5.32 am (90-second duration). All spells were stereotypical in nature. After sitting up from either stage N2 or stage N3 sleep, she exhibited up to 15 seconds of neck hyperextension with tonic extension of the right upper extremity, while emitting coarse respiratory and choking sounds in association with frank obstructive apneas (Figure 27.1). These events were followed by up to 30 seconds of generalized, low-amplitude clonic activity of all four extremities, and ended with loud, labored respirations, 2 minutes of postictal confusion and a subsequent return to sleep.

The EEG preceding some spells revealed an almost rhythmic slow, delta/theta brainwave pattern without frank sharp or spike discharges (suspected to have been obscured by significant movement artifact). As such, only one event was associated with a frank EEG abnormality, evidenced as poorly organized, postictal delta slow-wave activity (Figure 27.2).

A structural brain lesion was suggested by a temporally predominant, relative paucity of spindle and vertex sharp activity from the left hemisphere on the sleep EEG. There were also intermittent slow-wave discharges from this same region that occurred without evidence of frank epileptiform activity. An MRI of the brain and brainstem was normal.

From the clinical description of the spells, the familial history of sleepwalking and the PSG results, the pediatric neurologist determined that the patient was suffering from both processes: a common parasomnia (sleepwalking) and nocturnal seizures.

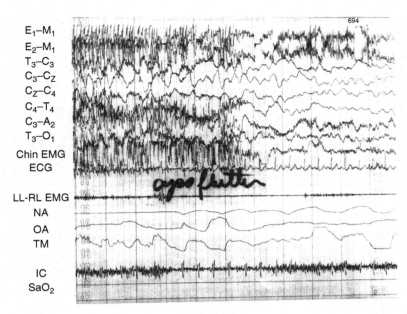

Figure 27.2 Abnormal postictal EEG. One of the patient's seven nocturnal events, described as a classic focal onset seizure with secondary generalization. The EEG shows poorly organized delta slow-wave activity, which was clinically associated with postictal confusion. Given the clinical concern for active seizure, the technician ran this segment of the PSG tracing at the standard EEG paper speed of 30 mm/s (rather than the standard PSG recording speed of 10 mm/s) to allow a clearer definition of the classic EEG seizure pattern. LL, left leg; RL, right leg; NA, nasal airflow; OA, oral airflow; TM, thoracic movement; IC, intercostal. (Reproduced with permission from Figure 9, in Dyken *et al.*, 2001.)

Diagnosis

The combination of PSG and clinical history led to a diagnosis of both somnambulism (sleepwalking) and seizure disorder. The PSG results unequivocally documented nocturnal seizures, while the history provided elements strongly suggesting somnambulism as a concomitant diagnosis. Nevertheless, the possibility that her sleepwalking episodes were actually representative of partial complex seizures or prolonged postictal states cannot be ruled out given the relative limitations of the evaluation.

Follow-up

After the PSG, the patient was initially treated with divided doses of valproic acid with the larger dose being given in the evening to address the nocturnal nature of the spells, and gradually being increased to 250 mg PO TID. At a 6-month follow-up, she was described as happy and doing well in school. She had a reduction in the frequency, duration and overall severity (in regard to the relatively violent nature) of nocturnal spells, with no sleepwalking for 3 consecutive months. Seizure-like activity now occurred only when she was overly tired. A trough valproic acid level was 89.7 in association with a relatively low total white blood cell count. No medication side effects were appreciated. She was subsequently found to have inherited the tendency for microcytic anemia from her father and was diagnosed with a two-gene deletion beta-thalassemia trait (beta-thalassemia minor). She was recommended to have any future potential child-bearing partners screened for alpha-thalassemia.

Within a year of her PSG diagnosis, the relatively early onset of menses at the age of 9 years was associated with a tendency for perimenstrual nocturnal seizures and a single flurry of daytime seizures. Over one 24-hour period, while awake, she experienced a series of ten seizures that involved stiffening of the right upper and lower extremities followed by tonic/clonic activity lasting less than 30 seconds. There was no reported aura or prolonged postictal state. The examination by her neurologist, performed within 3 days of the daytime seizures, revealed a new tendency for her to hold the right arm in flexion while walking. The mild lateralizing signs were considered to be unusual postictal residual (a Todd's-like paresis). Cognitively, however, the patient was doing well in a 5th-grade "gifted" program.

A follow-up evaluation performed 3 months later revealed that she continued to have one to three perimenstrual seizures per month and a tendency to favor the right leg when walking on her heels or toes. The use of a carbonic anhydrase inhibitor around the time of her monthly period was taken under consideration.

At the age of 11 (2 years postdiagnosis), she was having a maximum of four perimenstrual nocturnal seizures per month, usually between midnight and 3 am, aggravated by sleep deprivation. The examination showed that she had relatively slow rapid alternating movements and reduced fine finger coordination in the right hand.

At the age of 12 (3.5 years postdiagnosis), she reported an improvement in seizure control while taking diphenylhydantoin (100 mg QAM and 150 mg QPM), with only rare seizures that were precipitated by sleep deprivation or by missing a dose of her anticonvulsant. She continued to do well in school and participated in extracurricular activities. The neurological examination by this time had normalized. In addition, transient gum hypertrophy was controlled through routine dental care.

At the age of 15 (6.5 years postdiagnosis), the combination of diphenylhydantoin (200 mg QPM) and lamotrigine (300 mg BID) resulted in a seizure-free period of greater than 6 months. This improvement in seizure control and the paucity of daytime events allowed her to eventually apply for a driver's license as permitted by her state regulations.

By the age of 21 (12.5 years postdiagnosis), she had only an occasional perimenstrual episode (sleep terrors and sleeptalking) while taking lamotrigine 300 mg BID. When sleep deprived, she reported up to two "auras" per week, where she woke up with a nervous feeling in her stomach that lasted less than 15 seconds. By this time, the patient had earned a degree in graphic arts and was active in the martial arts.

At 27 years of age (18 years postdiagnosis), she appeared as an alert, oriented and well-groomed adult with fluid speech and a non-focal neurological examination. She had not experienced a daytime seizure for 9 years or a nocturnal seizure for over 2 years while taking lamotrigine 250 mg BID. Her medication had been reduced to successfully address dose-related diplopia. At this time, her Department of Transportation renewal to drive was provided by her epileptologist (as mandated for her specific line of employment). As she was now expressing an interest in child bearing, folate 1 mg per day was recommended to address potential teratogenicity issues of the anticonvulsant therapy. Also, a repeat recommendation was made to have any potential child-bearing partners screened for alpha-thalassemia given her previous diagnosis of beta-thalassemia.

General remarks

There is an extensive body of literature that addresses the formal definition of seizure when utilizing a minimum 16-channel sleep/wake EEG. Nevertheless, when attempting to differentiate a nocturnal seizure from a parasomnia, there are significant confounding issues associated with the diagnostic accuracy of PSG. Dyken *et al.* (2001) have referred to this difficulty as the "interference pattern."

The EEG concomitants of an active seizure have classically included generalized depression or slowing, rhythmic slow-wave or spike/polyspike and wave activity that can occur immediately prior to or during an event, and postictal slowing or depression frequently following a spell. Minimal or no ictal abnormalities can occur during some simple partial, myoclonic, and frontal lobe seizures. No EEG changes are appreciated in up to 5–10% of partial complex seizures.

In the sleep laboratory, these problems can be exacerbated by the relatively minimalist EEG montage routinely used in the standard PSG study, which may not include the brain area of primary epileptiform discharge. Moreover, short-lived ictal EEG changes are often obscured by EMG movement artifacts. In addition, the standard PSG recording speed of 10 mm/s has a compressing effect that can obscure subtle EEG abnormalities that might otherwise go unnoticed during a rapid review of extensive PSG data.

In some cases with a deep-seated cortical seizure focus, the limited PSG montage and combined effects of EEG compression and high-amplitude semi-rhythmic EMG artifacts can suggest the diagnosis of a parasomnia. This is especially true in disorders of arousal from NREM sleep, including confusional arousals, sleepwalking and sleep terrors. These disorders are strongly associated with the high-amplitude delta slow-wave activity of stage N3 sleep and behaviors that at times can simulate seizures.

This case study emphasizes that the clear differentiation between a nocturnal seizure and parasomnia is often difficult. The waking EEG and neurological examination can be normal and there are intrinsic limitations of the standard PSG. For this patient, the attended PSG study allowed immediate clinical observation and examination during the events of concern. This allowed a more focused and detailed analysis of the behaviors captured on video and their electrographic correlates. As such, we were able to recognize classic seizures of focal onset with secondary generalization, followed by a period of postictal confusion associated with subtle but unequivocal postictal EEG slow-wave activity (Figures 27.1 and 27.2).

Pearls and gold

Clear differentiation between a nocturnal seizure and parasomnia is often difficult.

The waking EEG and neurological examination can be normal and there are intrinsic limitations of the standard PSG.

In the sleep laboratory, diagnostic problems can be exacerbated by the relatively minimalist EEG montage routinely used in the standard PSG study, which may not include the brain area of primary epileptiform discharge.

The EEG concomitants of an active seizure have classically included generalized depression or slowing, rhythmic slow-wave or spike/polyspike and wave activity that can occur immediately prior to or during an event, and postictal slowing or depression frequently following a spell.

No EEG changes are appreciated in up to 5–10% of partial complex seizures.

Video recording and response to treatment aid in making a diagnosis of probability, if not of certainty.

SUGGESTED READING

HISTORICAL

Gastaut H, Broughton R. *Epileptic Seizures.* Springfield, Illinois: Charles C Thomas; 1972.

REVIEW

Dyken ME, Yamada T, Lin-Dyken DC. Polysomnographic assessment of spells in sleep: nocturnal seizures versus parasomnias. *Semin Neurol* 2001; **21**: 377–90.

GENERAL

AASM (American Academy of Sleep Medicine). *International Classification of Sleep Disorders,* 2nd edn.: *Diagnostic and Coding Manual.* Westchester, Illinois: American Academy of Sleep Medicine, 2005.

Klass DW. Electroencehalographic mechanisms of complex partial seizures. In: Penry JK, Daly DD, eds. *Complex Partial Seizures and Their Treatment.* New York: Raven Press; 1975: 113–40.

Klass DW, Espinosa RE, Fischer-Williams M. Analysis of concurrent electroencephalographic and clinical events occurring sequentially during partial seizures [Abstract]. *Electroencephalogr Clin Neurophysiol* 1973; **34**: 728.

Seizure, parasomnia or behavioral disorder?

Mark Eric Dyken and Deborah C. Lin-Dyken

Clinical history

A 10-year-old girl, who lived with her paternal grandmother as her divorced parents had recently failed an attempt at reconciliation, presented to a pediatric neurology clinic with a 3-week history of nocturnal and diurnal spells. At night, she woke from sleep screaming and thrashing, and after 20 seconds would quickly return to sleep. She also experienced up to five unprovoked 20-second spells per day during which she would suddenly become tense and disoriented with facial flushing and right-eye twitching, after which she was appropriately responsive, but appeared unsteady on her feet and reported either a headache or a stomachache. The frequency of these events caused her to miss many days of school.

She also had a 5-year history of daily spells associated with the sudden onset of paresthesia in the left arm, lasting up to 30 seconds, which were followed by right-sided headaches. These events were without aura, change in level of consciousness or a clear postictal state.

The patient was the product of an uncomplicated pregnancy, had reached developmental milestones in a normal fashion and was not on any medications. Her parents had divorced 2 years previously. She had required counseling at the age of 5 years for vivid memories of being molested by a babysitter at the age of 3 and of her father beating her mother and brother at the age of 4. The family history revealed bipolar affective disorder in her mother and attention deficit hyperactivity disorder and febrile seizures in her younger brother.

Examination

The patient appeared alert, cooperative and in no distress. Her vital signs, anthropometric data (weight 38.0 kg, head circumference 52.5 cm) and general examinations were unremarkable. The neurological examination revealed a patchy decrease to light touch in the left arm.

Case Studies in Sleep Neurology: Common and Uncommon Presentations, ed. A. Culebras. Published by Cambridge University Press. © Cambridge University Press 2010.

Special studies

An awake EEG and continuous nocturnal video-EEG were carried out.

Question

Are the spells seizures or parasomnia events?

Results of studies

The EEG in the waking state was normal.

Continuous video-EEG with telemetry captured 40 stereotypical spells throughout the night where the patient would suddenly wake up with a frightened appearance and loudly call for "Daddy" (who was present throughout the study), while crouching on her hands and knees. She would then cling to her father, while apparently at her normal waking level of cognition, after which she would return to sleep (Figure 28.1). Every spell occurred during stage N2 sleep, with the exception of one that arose from REM sleep. Obvious EEG abnormalities were not appreciated during most spells (Figure 28.2). One event was associated with rhythmic, right frontal theta EEG activity, while another was followed by right hemispheric delta slow-wave activity (Figure 28.2).

Diagnosis

The combination of the observed behavior and EEG findings suggested nocturnal frontal lobe epilepsy (NFLE), whereas the daytime events were considered to be panic attacks.

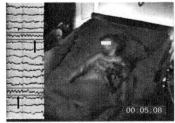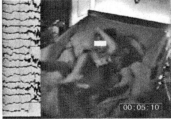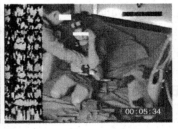

Figure 28.1 Of the 40 stereotypical spells captured during a 10-year-old girl's sleep video-EEG, only one showed rhythmic theta activity from the right frontal region (as shown by the arrows in the EEG channels enclosed by the rectangular boxes in the left-hand picture) prior to a clinical spell, which was characterized by a sudden frightened awakening and yelling for "Daddy" (middle picture), and followed by crouching on bended hands and knees and subsequently (right-hand picture) clutching her father.

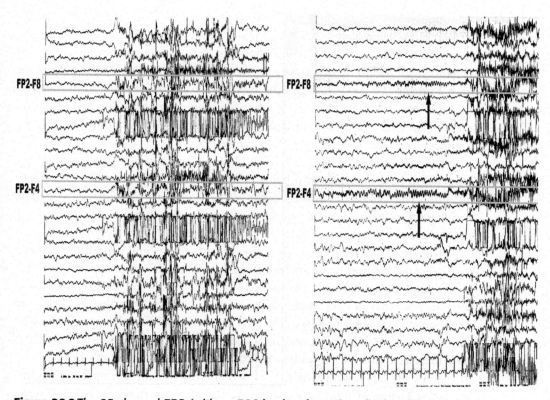

Figure 28.2 The 25-channel EEG (with an ECG lead and a review display of 10 mm/s) of a 10-year-old girl during one of her stereotypical nocturnal spells from sleep associated with fear shows no appreciable abnormalities before, during or after a brief clinical event (including the EEG channels from the right frontal region as delineated by the gray rectangular boxes in the left-hand picture). Of the 40 stereotypical spells captured, only one showed rhythmic theta activity from the right frontal region (as shown by the arrows in the EEG channels that are enclosed by the rectangular boxes in the right-hand picture) immediately prior to a clinical spell characterized by frightened loud vocalizations and hypermotor activity that otherwise superficially could mimic a parasomnia or behavioral disorder. (Modified with permission from Figures 6 and 7, in Dyken *et al.*, 2001).

Follow-up

The patient was treated with carbamazepine (200 mg BID) for NFLE and entered formal counseling with behavior modification techniques for daytime panic attacks. At 1 month follow-up, the nocturnal spells had resolved. The suspected behavioral problems, which were worse at home than at school, persisted as episodes of defiance.

Although the neurological examination had normalized with treatment, the EEG findings demanded an MRI study of the brain to rule out a focal right frontal lesion. The MRI revealed a lesion that was 2 cm in diameter, which did not enhance with gadolinium and was hypodense on T1 imaging and hyperintense on T2 imaging. It was located in the inferior left cerebellar tonsil and extended into the vermis with minimal mass effect (without edema) causing mild deformation of the fourth ventricle without hydrocephalus. Within a month, the tumor, a pilocytic astrocytoma, was completely resected.

Six months after the diagnosis of NFLE and panic attacks, the patient was reported to have intermittent tingling in the left hand and foot and a "negative" attitude. The cerebellar lesion on the other hand was considered to be an incidental finding, which did not seem to be related to her NFLE or behavioral problems.

At the age of 11, one year after the diagnosis of seizures and panic attacks, there had been no recurrence of nocturnal spells and therefore carbamazepine was tapered and discontinued. At the age of 13 (after 2 years off carbamazepine), there was no recurrence of nocturnal seizures or panic attacks. Nevertheless, there was persistence of episodes of paresthesia that now involved the left upper and lower extremities, several of which now occurred upon awakening. Their duration had also increased from 15 minutes to lasting throughout most of the day. On occasions, her left fingers would also involuntarily twitch, leaving her with the subjective feeling of mild hand weakness. She also reported that twice a week, upon quickly rising from sleep, her vision would go black for a few seconds.

A follow-up brain MRI was unremarkable and without evidence of tumor recurrence. A formal EEG showed intermittent low-voltage spike discharges from the right temporal area, mostly in sleep. This was felt to be consistent with a focal seizure tendency. The examination now showed a very mild left hemiparetic gait and three beats of right ankle clonus. The neurologist recommended a gradual increase in carbamazepine to 200 mg TID for recurrent simple partial seizures.

At the age of 14, 4 years after the initial diagnosis of seizures and panic attacks, the patient had not reinstated the use of carbamazepine and continued to have left hemibody paresthesias. Nevertheless, she now had a non-focal neurological examination, and a repeat MRI of the brain was found to be unremarkable.

At 17 years, 7 years after the initial diagnosis of seizure and panic attacks, the patient was admitted to the hospital with suicidal ideation with planning, after she had recently broken up with a boyfriend, fought with a friend in school (leading to a 3-day suspension) and verbally and physically assaulted her father and stepmother. The father indicated that the patient's biological mother had exhibited similar behavioral problems. The patient was subsequently diagnosed with depression and a borderline personality disorder.

At the age of 19, 9 years after the initial diagnosis of seizure and panic disorder, the patient was diagnosed with a recurrence of panic attacks that now occurred primarily at night in association with dyspnea, dizziness and tingling and numbness of all four extremities. An MRI of the brain at that time was unremarkable. She was again admitted to the hospital with depression and suicidal ideation, after which she was lost to follow-up.

General remarks

Nocturnal frontal lobe epilepsy is a heterogeneous disorder that affects all age groups, with an estimated mean age of onset of 14 ± 10 years, and is characterized by seizures that occur either exclusively or predominately during sleep, with approximately 34% reporting occasional seizures (similar to their sleep seizures) during daytime wakefulness. The neurological examination has been reported to be normal in up to 92% of cases. Although there are no major clinical differences between the sporadic and the autosomal dominantly inherited form of NFLE, concomitant diurnal behavioral disturbances including impulsivity, aggression and hyperactivity have been reported in some forms of NFLE in relation to mutations of the subunits of the nicotinic acetylcholine receptor.

Nocturnal frontal lobe epilepsy is generally associated with relatively brief hypermotor seizures, often with marked autonomic activation, that can appear as paroxysmal nocturnal dystonia, episodic nocturnal wanderings or as frequent stereotypical arousals with emotive vocalizations and bending and rocking of the body that often suggest an underlying parasomnia or behavioral event. The firm diagnosis is also complicated by the fact that the EEG is often normal. In one large study of 100 consecutively encountered patients with NFLE, 55% of patients had normal interictal awake EEGs, 51% of subjects had unremarkable interictal sleep studies and 44% had normal ictal polysomnographic evaluations (although the EEG reading was frequently masked by muscle or clouded by sleep-related phenomena).

Tao et al. (2005, 2007) have shown that a certain degree of cerebral activation, which is dependent on the cerebral source area and synchrony of electrical discharge from the epileptiform focus, is required to generate a recordable scalp EEG ictal pattern. Their studies focused on identifying the source area for spikes originating from the antero- and inferolateral temporal cortex, as these spike voltage fields are primarily radial in orientation and provide the highest level of EEG detectability. Using simultaneous recordings from 26 channels of EEG with subtemporal supplementary electrodes and 46–96 channels of intracranial EEG recordings (in candidates preparing for possible temporal lobe epilepsy surgery), they estimated that at least $10–20 \, cm^2$ of synchronously activated gyral cortex is generally needed for detection of spike activity (indicative of seizure potential) by scalp surface EEG electrodes. The authors believed that their results defined the lower limit of source area for scalp spikes, as other extratemporal sources with tangential voltage fields would require an even larger area to result in recognizable scalp EEG potentials. This has been used by some experts to explain why a deep-seated frontal lobe seizure focus with a tangentially oriented voltage field in a patient with NFLE might not routinely produce an EEG abnormality.

In addition, imaging studies generally do not routinely provide evidence of frontal lobe abnormality in NFLE. In some studies, focal abnormalities on brain CT and MRI have been reported in only 12% of patients. In anecdotal reports, a single patient with sporadic NFLE was shown to have anterior cingulate hyper-perfusion using ictal single-photon-emission CT (SPECT), whereas in two cases of autosomal dominant NFLE, SPECT has respectively shown mesial frontal and orbitofrontal/frontopolar hyperperfusion (anteroinferior frontal lobe hypometabolism using [^{18}F]fluorodeoxyglucose positron emission tomography was also shown in one of these cases).

In one study, carbamazepine abolished all seizures in approximately 20% of cases. A significant reduction in seizure activity by at least 50% was reported in another 48% of the patients in this same study. The neuropsychological profile in NFLE has not been well studied. Some groups have reported no obvious intellectual problems in these patients, while several anecdotal reports and small case studies have documented individuals with cognitive and adaptive disabilities and behavioral problems. Some experts believe that behavioral disturbances and cognitive problems associate particularly with mutations within the subunits of the nicotinic acetylcholine receptor. Their concern is that more subtle deficits may be overlooked in any given case, and as such they believe this issue is deserving of specific study in the future.

The present case study emphasizes that the clear differentiation between NFLE, parasomnias and behavioral disorders is often difficult, as in any given patient the neurological examination, EEG and brain imaging studies can all be normal. As such, the routine diagnosis of NFLE is generally dependent upon the semiological appearance of spells that are similar to those reported historically by individuals with known orbitofrontal and mesial frontal lobe lesions. In this case, a focused and detailed analysis of nocturnal stereotypical behaviors captured during continuous, prolonged video-EEG monitoring using an extended montage allowed us to document unequivocal epileptiform discharge, confirming the diagnosis of NFLE (Figures 28.1 and 28.2). Nevertheless, the significant behavioral concomitants associated with her clinical presentation throughout years of long-term follow-up routinely raised concern regarding the adequacy of her seizure control.

Pearls and gold

The diagnosis of NFLE is generally dependent upon the semiological appearance of spells that are similar to those reported historically by individuals with known orbitofrontal and mesial frontal lobe lesions.

The clear differentiation between NFLE, parasomnias and behavioral disorders is often difficult, as in any given patient the neurological examination, EEG and brain imaging studies can all be normal.

SUGGESTED READING

Dyken ME, Yamada T, Lin-Dyken DC. Polysomnographic assessment of spells in sleep: nocturnal seizures versus parasomnias. *Semin Neurol* 2001; **21**: 377–90.

Provini F, Plazzi G, Tinuper P, *et al.* Nocturnal frontal lobe epilepsy. A clinical and polygraphic overview of 100 consecutive cases. *Brain* 1999; **122**: 1017–31.

Ryvlin P, Rheims S, Risse G. Nocturnal frontal lobe epilepsy. *Epilepsia* 2006; **47**: 83–6.

Tao JX, Ray A, Hawes-Ebersole S, *et al.* Intracranial EEG substrates of scalp EEG interictal spikes. *Epilepsia* 2005; **46**: 669–76.

Tao JX, Baldwin M, Ray A, *et al.* The impact of cerebral source area and synchrony on recording scalp electroencephalography ictal patterns. *Epilepsia* 2007; **48**: 2167–76.

Sounds of choking at night

Bradley V. Vaughn and Chon Lee

Clinical history

SB was a 7-year-old girl brought to her physician for episodes that occurred soon
after going to bed. With each event, the mother heard an unusual sound of lip
smacking and choking coming from the child's bedroom. The child would awaken
lightly crying, drooling and unable to speak and with the right side of her face
twitching. The episodes lasted approximately 60–90 seconds in duration. Afterwards,
her right face would droop and she had difficulty talking. The patient would go back
to bed and sleep through the remaining portion of the night. The patient had suffered
four events since the start, 3 months prior to her clinic visit. She had no symptoms of
daytime sleepiness, insomnia, sleepwalking or excessive movement at night.

The patient was born at term and demonstrated normal development. She was
a good student in home schooling at the first-grade level and well adjusted in her
play environment. At 2 years of age, she had lymphadenopathy and underwent
lymph node biopsy, the results of which were normal. She had seasonal allergies
for which she was given allergy shots. Her mother had migraines and there was no
family history of sleep disorders, seizures or epilepsy.

Examination

SB was a well-appearing child with appropriate growth. Her general examination
was normal. She was alert and had normal cognition. Her cranial nerves ware intact,
and motor tone, bulk and strength were normal, movements were coordinated,
sensation was intact to all modalities, reflexes were 2+ and symmetric, and gait was
normal including tandem gait.

Special studies

Due to the stereotypic events, the patient underwent an MRI of her brain and
sleep-deprived EEG.

Case Studies in Sleep Neurology: Common and Uncommon Presentations, ed. A. Culebras. Published by
Cambridge University Press. © Cambridge University Press 2010.

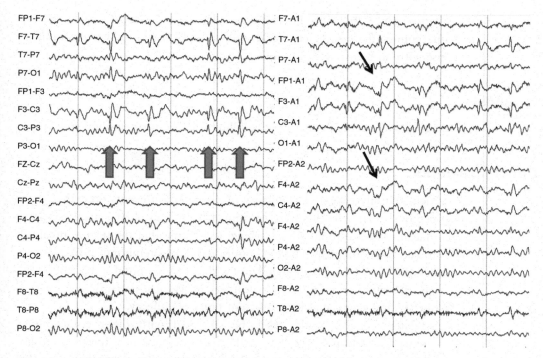

Figure 29.1 The figure shows centrotemporal spikes in drowsiness with both bipolar and referential montage. The panel on the left shows centrotemporal spikes on a "double banana" montage (blue arrows). The right panel shows a referential montage; the black arrows demonstrate the horizontal dipole and bifrontal positivity that occurs in classical benign epilepsy with centrotemporal spikes (BECTS) patients.

Question

Are these episodes parasomnias or seizure events?

Results of studies

The patient's MRI of the brain was normal. However, the sleep-deprived EEG showed left centrotemporal spikes greater than right that were more prominent in drowsiness and sleep (Figure 29.1).

Follow-up

After a long discussion with SB's parents, the family decided to wait to see if the events resolved without medication. Within 6 months, the patient was having more frequent events and the family was again offered a trial of anticonvulsant therapy to reduce the episodes. SB was started on low-dose regular-release carbamazepine (after a complete blood count was obtained) and had an excellent response with no recurrence of events.

Diagnosis

The diagnosis was benign epilepsy of childhood with centrotemporal spikes.

General remarks

The patient's family gave a clear history of stereotypical events occurring soon after sleep onset. These events were accompanied by typical ictal manifestations of hemifacial spasms, drooling and jerking, suggesting that the seizure involved the contralateral motor strip. The EEG findings of centrotemporal spikes in sleep supported the diagnosis of benign epilepsy with centrotemporal spikes (BECTS). Although, this child had the classical features of BECTS, patients may express similar behavioral events and have different types of epilepsy.

Sleep-related seizures could easily be confused with other parasomnias or psychiatric conditions, especially if the patients have no diurnal findings. The historical review from witnesses of the events may give cardinal clues to the etiology. These events have similar behavior each time, which is a key feature of epileptic seizures. The feature of stereotypic behavior points to a possible underlying epileptic disorder. Nocturnal seizures can produce a wide range of behaviors; thus, a clear description of the behaviors is paramount. The behavioral expression of the seizure depends upon the location of the seizure discharge. Nearly any behavior that can be produced by the brain can be exhibited as a seizure (Table 29.1). However, seizures are stereotypic, each seizure having similar behavior to the others for an individual. The frontal and temporal lobes are the most common sites for seizure foci, and these are areas more commonly involved in sleep-related epilepsies.

Seizures involving the frontal lobes may evoke tonic posturing, complex bizarre motor activity and even violent behavior. Temporal lobe seizures usually produce episodes of staring, psychic phenomena and some complex behaviors. Temporal and frontal lobe seizures can also evoke a wide range of autonomic symptoms, such as bradycardia, asystole, tachycardia, emesis and respiratory disturbances. Parietal onset seizures are more likely to evoke disturbances or distortion of sensory perception. Occipital lobe onset seizures are usually associated with visual phenomena, visual distortion or eye movement. Benign occipital epilepsy of childhood is frequently associated with nocturnal seizures, vomiting and headache and is frequently misdiagnosed as migraine. With the complexity of these

Table 29.1 Seizure-related behaviors

Seizure location	Possible behaviors (not limited to)
Frontal	Posturing of extremities, vocalization, rocking, turning, ambulation, sitting up, pelvic thrusting, gestural automatisms, jerking of face or extremities
Temporal	Staring, an absence of other activity, autonomic events, olfactory and auditory hallucinations, out-of-body and psychic experiences, oroalimentary automatisms, expressions of fear, rising epigastric sensation, belching
Parietal	Somatosensory events (tingling, electrical, wave-like, temperature change or numbness), feeling of movement in a portion of the body or vertigo, metamorphopsia
Occipital	Visual hallucinations (sparks, flashes or more formed images), hemianopsia, scotoma, visual distortion
Generalized	Whole-body stiffening or clonic jerking; myoclonus may involve the whole body or any portion of the body

behaviors, one can easily see an overlap in presentation among patients with seizures and parasomnias.

Following the seizure, patients are frequently confused and disoriented. The authors have recorded wandering behavior, pronounced violence, rhythmic movement, snoring and even psychosis as postictal events. The confusion may resolve over minutes or may only improve after the patient sleeps. Postictal somnolence is common and can make differentiating seizures from a parasomnia very difficult. The patient may also have postictal focal issues including numbness, speech problems or weakness, formerly known as Todd's paralysis. These findings may last minutes to hours.

To distinguish simple partial seizures from complex partial seizures, the patient must experience either loss of memory or impairment of consciousness. Amnesia indicates that both hippocampal structures were involved in the seizure event. If one hippocampus is not impaired during the seizure, patients will maintain memory. Patients without temporal lobe extension of their seizures can have retained memory for the events and therefore may have complex behaviors with retained memory. These patients are frequently mislabeled as having psychogenic disorders.

Several nocturnal seizure syndromes exist in both adults and children. Some of these have been designated as benign, while others are on a spectrum of disorders that have significant neurological consequences. One of the best examples includes BECTS. This disorder, formerly known as rolandic epilepsy, is on the spectrum of disorders including BECTS, Landau–Kleffner syndrome and continuous spike and wave in sleep (CSWS). Each of these has diagnostic criteria;

however, the latter two have long-term neurological sequelae. Another disorder similar to BECTS, benign occipital lobe epilepsy of childhood, raises a similar question relative to the issue of "benign."

Benign focal epilepsy with centrotemporal spikes or benign rolandic epilepsy, also known as BECTS, is a form of inherited nocturnal seizure. It occurs in children between 3 and 13 years of age and resolves by the age of 18. Patients typically present with episodes of hemifacial and body tonic activity, drooling and speech impairment. Occasionally, these patients have a generalized seizure. These events occur approximately 20 minutes to 2 hours after going to bed and last less then 5 minutes. An EEG usually demonstrates a high-amplitude spike with a scalloped secondary positive waveform in the centrotemporal region. These spikes are more frequent during drowsiness and sleep. As in this case, classical BECTS patients will show a horizontal dipole (combination of simultaneous negative and positive waves) with bifrontal positivity. Patients are neurologically normal and respond favorably to anticonvulsant medications. Some clinicians elect to withhold medication, as the seizures typically resolve during adolescence.

Benign nocturnal childhood occipital epilepsy or Panayiotopoulos syndrome was first described in 1989, and was originally characterized by the constellation of nocturnal seizures, tonic eye deviation and nocturnal vomiting typically starting in childhood and ending in adolescence. These nocturnal events usually arise between 4 and 12 years and resolve by the age of 16. The EEG demonstrates spike and slow-wave discharges in the occipital region and may include generalized discharges. Further descriptions have expanded the spectrum of clinical manifestations, demonstrating cases in which there is overlap with other focal idiopathic epilepsies such as benign rolandic epilepsy and other generalized epilepsy syndromes. Most of these patients respond favorably to medication. Landau–Kleffner syndrome, or acquired epileptic aphasia, does not typically result in obvious sleep complaints, but is hallmarked by a decline in language abilities. Children in the 3–9 years range develop verbal auditory agnosia and may be misdiagnosed as deaf. Patients may also develop behavioral abnormalities. Approximately 70% of patients have seizures, usually nocturnal, and most seizures are manifested by eye blinking, eye deviation, head drops or other automatisms. This syndrome, similar to BECTS, may be associated with a normal EEG during wakefulness and prominent spike and spike and wave discharges during sleep. The epileptiform discharges can be focal, bilateral and generalized, but are more common in the temporal, central and parietal regions. They can occur in runs and may cause fragmentation of sleep. The disorder is thought to represent a middle ground between BECTS and CSWS or electrical status epilepticus during sleep. Patients may show some improvement or slowing of the decline in verbal function with anticonvulsant medication.

Continuous spike and wave during sleep or electrical status epilepticus during sleep is characterized by near-continuous spike wave discharges during slow-wave sleep, focal or generalized seizures and neuropsychological decline. Children with this disorder may manifest nocturnal seizures and then have significant cognitive and psychological decline. Many of these children will have nocturnal and diurnal absence events along with focal motor and generalized tonic/clonic seizures. The EEG in sleep is the key to diagnosis. Near-continuous epileptiform activity replaces normal EEG features of sleep, but only one in five children has epileptiform activity when awake. Case reports have documented that some patients respond to levetiracetam therapy; however, prognosis is usually guarded.

Autosomal dominant nocturnal frontal lobe epilepsy (ADNFLE), previously known as hypnogenic paroxysmal dystonia or nocturnal paroxysmal dystonia (NPD), is characterized by repeated dystonic or dyskinetic episodes occurring at night. The movements can involve a single extremity or up to all four extremities and the neck. Occasionally, patients may vocalize and frequently recall the event. They typically occur out of NREM sleep and demonstrate two major forms: short duration (15–60 seconds) and long duration (up to 60 minutes). Patients may have multiple spells per night or may have clusters of spells with relatively quiescent periods. Nocturnal paroxysmal dystonia is considered to be a form of frontal lobe epilepsy. An Italian form of inherited nocturnal frontal lobe epilepsy (NFLE) has been described. This complex disorder may show episodes of nocturnal dystonia, paroxysmal arousals and nocturnal wandering. It is passed in an autosomal dominant pattern. The family history can be difficult to obtain, as the spells may not be recognized by or acknowledged to other family members. About one in four of these individuals will have daytime seizures. The EEG frequently demonstrates no epileptic changes during the spells, and daytime EEGs are normal. Patients may demonstrate any combination of nocturnal behaviors with few EEG changes. Most patients respond to anticonvulsant medication.

The Australian form of ADNFLE has been linked to chromosome 20q13.2 to the CHRNA4 gene. An abnormality of the neuronal nicotinic acetylcholine receptor subunits has been found in association with this disorder. Although augmentation of acetylcholine does not appear to alter the frequency or intensity of the seizures, nicotine may influence some function of select receptor abnormalities.

Epileptic-based myoclonus can occur soon after awakening in myoclonic epilepsy. The rapid jerk of myoclonus can involve any region of the body. Myoclonus associated with the awakening epilepsies frequently occurs soon after arousal. The jerks can occur as single events or in a rapid succession. Sleep deprivation will exacerbate the events. They should be differentiated from hypnic jerks, which occur at sleep onset and periodic limb movements of sleep (PLMS), which occur mostly during NREM sleep.

All patients with suspected nocturnal seizures should have a complete neurological examination and should undergo MRI investigation of the brain and an EEG during sleep. In cases of evident neurological decline, an overnight EEG recording is an option to evaluate for CSWS. Patients should be followed for frequency of events, response to medication and, if needed, consideration for further evaluation by an epilepsy specialist.

Pearls and gold

Sleep-related seizures can easily be confused with other parasomnias or psychiatric conditions, especially if the patients have no diurnal findings.

The feature of stereotypic behavior points to a possible underlying epileptic disorder.

The behavioral expression of the seizure depends upon the location of the seizure discharge.

Amnesia indicates that both hippocampal structures were involved in the seizure event; if one hippocampus is not impaired during the seizure, patients can maintain memory.

All patients with suspected nocturnal seizures should have a complete neurological examination and should undergo MRI investigation of the brain and an EEG during sleep.

SUGGESTED READING

HISTORICAL

Beaussart M. Benign epilepsy of childhood with rolandic (centrotemporal) paroxysmal foci. *Epilepsia* 1972; **13**: 795–811.

REVIEWS

Capovilla G, Striano P, Beccaria F. Changes in Panayiotopoulos syndrome over time. *Epilepsia* 2009; **50** (Suppl. 5): S45–S8.

Gobbi G, Boni A, Filippini M. The spectrum of idiopathic Rolandic epilepsy syndromes and idiopathic occipital epilepsies: from the benign to the disabling. *Epilepsia* 2006; **47** (Suppl. 2): S62–S6.

Kramer U. Atypical presentations of benign childhood epilepsy with centrotemporal spikes: a review. *J Child Neurol* 2008; **23**: 785–90.

Nickels K, Wirrell E. Electrical status epilepticus in sleep. *Semin Pediatr Neurol* 2008; **15**: 50–60.

GENERAL

Son CD, Moss FJ, Cohen BN, Lester HA. Nicotine normalizes intracellular subunit stoichiometry of nicotinic receptors carrying mutations linked to autosomal dominant nocturnal frontal lobe epilepsy. *Mol Pharmacol* 2009; **75**: 1137–48.

Zacconi M, Ferini-Strambi L. NREM parasomnias: arousals and differentiation from nocturnal frontal lobe epilepsy. *Clin Neurophysiol* 2000; **111** (Suppl. 2): S129–S35.

Case 30

Fighting in sleep

Lynn V. Kataria and Bradley V. Vaughn

Clinical history

Mr J. was a 42-year-old man who presented with a 2-year history of events of yelling and fighting in his sleep that were brought to his attention by his wife. She described the events as him yelling out and then striking the headboard repetitively with his fist. The events were typically in the first half of the night and lasted for approximately 10–30 seconds after which he resumed sleep. Mr J. had no memory of the events and he was initially unsure that the events had really happened until he awoke with a bruised hand. He denied any associated dream recall or feeling of threat. Mrs J. began sleeping in a separate bed due to concern that she might be injured. The morning following an event, Mr J. felt mildly tired, but had no other daytime complaints. Initially, the events occurred approximately every 2 months, but later the frequency was once per week. His wife noted that Mr J. was under significant stress at work and she was concerned that these events were related. On more specific questioning, his wife noted that the patient's eyes were closed during the events. A loud noise or a sudden arousal did not provoke the events. Otherwise, the patient was a relatively quiet sleeper and did not snore. She denied that he had leg kicking, thrashing or other nighttime episodes. During the daytime, the patient denied sleepiness or symptoms suggestive of cataplexy, sleep paralysis or seizures. There was no history of sleepwalking or night terror events during childhood or adolescence.

The patient had a history of mild hypertension for which he was receiving hydrochlorothiazide. His father had a history of coronary artery disease and his brother had sleepwalking as a child. The patient denied tobacco use and admitted only rare alcohol use, which was not associated with the nocturnal events. In a review of systems, the patient described lower libido; all other systems were negative.

Case Studies in Sleep Neurology: Common and Uncommon Presentations, ed. A. Culebras. Published by Cambridge University Press. © Cambridge University Press 2010.

Examination

The patient was a normal-appearing middle-aged male with a heart rate of 82 bpm, respiratory rate of 16 breaths per minute, blood pressure of 126/84 mmHg and weight of 81 kg. The remaining areas of his general and neurological examinations were normal.

Special studies

Given the event description, the patient underwent a sleep-deprived EEG followed by video-EEG monitoring. The patient also had an MRI of the brain.

Question

What is the etiology of these nocturnal events?

Follow-up

After the initial visit, the patient was advised to keep a calendar of events and an account of potential aggravators such as sleep deprivation, alcohol and caffeine use or stress levels for the day prior to the event. His wife was asked to write a description of the episodes she witnessed and whether she heard snoring.

Results of studies

The diary showed that the events occurred approximately once per week and the behavior recorded was similar to Mrs J.'s initial description. A sleep-deprived EEG was normal; however, he did not fall asleep during the recording. Subsequently, the patient underwent video-EEG monitoring. After 5 days of recording, two events were captured. The behavior of the first event consisted of a brief vocalization followed by the left arm being punched above the patient's head with some bicycling movements of the legs. There was no concurrent change in the EEG. The second video event was characterized by similar vocalization and movement of the left arm with more prominent bicycling of the legs. This episode lasted approximately 20 seconds; widespread rhythmical slowing followed by a clear epileptiform rhythm across the frontal regions was present prior to the movement (Figure 30.1).

Diagnosis

Given these results, the specialist made a diagnosis of focal-onset epilepsy and pursued an MRI of the brain. The imaging study was within normal limits.

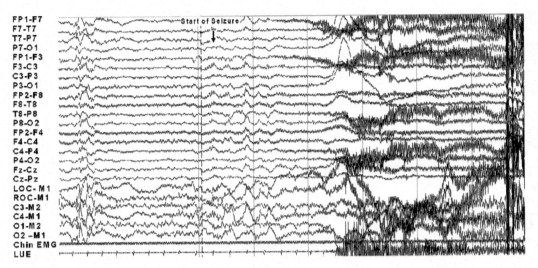

Figure 30.1 The combined EEG and polysomnographic recording demonstrates the onset of seizure activity as rhythmical slow waves followed by faster activity in the frontal regions several seconds prior to the behavioral event. LUE, left upper extremity.

The patient was subsequently started on regular-release carbamazepine with a higher dose in the evening. After adjustment of the medication, the patient had complete resolution of his nocturnal events.

General remarks

Nearly 3% of adults and 15% of children have nocturnal events. Diagnosing nocturnal events can be an arduous task, even for the most skilled clinicians. However, diligence is important, as differentiating their etiology may herald other underlying health issues. Nocturnal events can be related to NREM-sleep parasomnias, REM-sleep parasomnias, psychiatric disorders, neurological disorders and medical disorders. Key historical and examination features may distinguish the types of events (Table 30.1). When evaluating patients presenting with symptoms of nocturnal episodic activity, it is critical to obtain a clear history from a witness. Important questions to ask include the patient's level of consciousness, the duration of the episode, time of the events, frequency of events, memory or dream recall, associated motor behaviors and the similarity of behaviors in serial events (stereotypical).

Parasomnias are undesirable physical and mental phenomena that occur during sleep and sleep/wake transitions. The most common NREM parasomnias

Table 30.1 Distinguishing features of nocturnal events

Feature	Disorders of arousal	REM-sleep behavior disorder	Nocturnal seizures	Psychiatric disorders
Time of night	First third of night	Latter half of sleep period during REM	Variable	Variable
Eye opening	Yes	No	No	Yes
Stereotypic movements	No	No	Yes	No
Memory	Usually partial or no memory	Vivid dream recall	Variable	Variable
Duration	Minutes	Seconds to minutes	Minutes	Minutes to hours
Frequency	One to three events per night	Nightly minor events	Variable	Variable
Age of onset	Childhood or adolescence	Usually adulthood	Any time	Any time
Polysomnography findings	Arousal from slow-wave sleep with potential to continue slowing	Excessive EMG activity in REM	Epileptiform activity	Wake state prior to the event

are the disorders of arousal. These events characteristically occur as a partial awakening from stage N3 sleep. They present as a mixture of sleep and wake states such that part of the brain is in slow-wave sleep while another part is awake. Disorders of arousal include sleepwalking, sleep terrors (night terrors or *pavor nocturnus*) and confusional arousals. There is full or partial amnesia for the event, occurrence in the first half of the night, non-stereotypic movements, open eyes and possible provocation by situations that cause arousal or increase slow-wave sleep. Most events last less than 3 minutes, but some can be prolonged. As defined by ICSD-2 (AASM, 2005), sleepwalking consists of complex coordinated motor behaviors, including standing and walking with the persistence of sleep. If patients are interrupted during the episode, they can exhibit a variety of behaviors from no response to aggressive and violent behavior. Sleepwalking is more common in childhood; most adults who present with sleepwalking had events as a child. Sleep terrors are hallmarked by a piercing scream coupled with the appearance of intense fear and signs of autonomic alteration such as profuse perspiration. Children are often inconsolable, and when caregivers attempt to console them, symptoms may worsen. Confusional arousals are characterized by arousals from sleep with inappropriate behavior. They occur as part of an awakening, and the patient may exhibit a variety of behaviors from relatively innocuous actions to disorientation and aggression. Confusional arousals tend to occur in children and young adults, especially after sleep deprivation.

These events are rarely captured in the sleep laboratory. On polysomnography (PSG), EEG patterns in NREM parasomnias exhibit a continuation of slowing into the arousal, tachycardia prior to the arousal and sometimes hypersynchronous delta waves. The last are not limited to parasomnias. However, there are often movement artifacts, which can make EEG interpretation difficult. More recent work by Pilon *et al.* (2008) suggests that a combination of sleep deprivation, sleeping at times when typically awake and a provocative noise presented in slow-wave sleep may elicit an event.

Once the diagnosis of disorder of arousal is established, treatment includes avoiding situations that increase slow-wave sleep, reducing potential arousals and promoting safety. Avoiding sleep deprivation reduces the risk of slow-wave sleep rebound and thus decreases the opportunity of recurrence of events. Patients should also reduce factors that potentially induce arousals such as light, excessive noise, stressors and multiple bed partners (children, pets), as well as treating disorders that cause arousal. If a patient exhibits symptoms of nocturia, pain or dyspnea at night, treating the underlying problem may decrease events. Obstructive sleep apnea (OSA) may also provoke NREM parasomnias by increasing the number of arousals. Appropriate treatment of sleep apnea in patients with an underlying disorder of arousal has been shown to reduce the frequency of events. Patients must be questioned regarding symptoms of sleep apnea. Safety is also paramount. When confronted with a patient that may be exhibiting a disorder of arousal, it is important to intervene. If the patient or someone else is at risk of injury, one should lead the patient back into bed to prevent further injury. Additional measures such as placing the mattress on the floor, removing all sharp or dangerous objects and placing a barrier in front of windows should be implemented. Locked doors and windows and moving the bedroom to the ground floor may reduce the risk of injury. Pharmacotherapy is initiated when events are violent, associated with injurious behavior to self or others, or when secondary manifestations result in excessive daytime sleepiness (EDS) or weight gain. Clonazapem 0.5–2 mg or diazepam 5 mg given before bedtime are the initial drugs of choice, but studies are limited. Both of these agents aim to suppress arousals rather than suppressing slow-wave sleep.

REM-sleep parasomnias include REM-sleep behavior disorder (RBD), nightmares, sleep paralysis, cataplexy and terrifying hypnagogic hallucinations. Nightmares and RBD are more applicable to this case. Nightmares are vivid, distressing dreams, more common in the latter half of the night and often associated with fear. Unlike RBD, nightmares have no motor manifestations associated with the dream. In contrast, patients with RBD act out their dreams due to a loss of the REM-sleep-associated atonia. Often, these events are violent and bed partners are frequently injured. Patients with RBD exhibit punching, kicking and screaming during the episodes, but the eyes are closed. Patients with RBD have dream recall for the event and the movements correlate with the dream content. Patients can have multiple episodes per night, but most last seconds to minutes. Patients rarely leave the bedroom during the event. Pathophysiologically, RBD represents a structural or chemical disruption of the mechanism for atonia during REM sleep. REM-sleep behavior disorder can occur acutely with the use of selective serotonin reuptake inhibitors (SSRIs), tricyclic antidepressants, norepin-ephrine reuptake blockers, neuroleptics and alcohol withdrawal. An MRI of the brain is helpful for evaluating structural etiologies such as stroke, tumor or demyelinating lesions. Many patients develop signs of Parkinsonism or other synucleinopathies, and therefore careful neurological evaluation is required. The key to diagnosis is excessive muscle activity during REM sleep by PSG recording of several muscle groups including the wrist extensors. As with all nocturnal events, safety is paramount. The bed partner should sleep in a separate room and sharp objects should not be near the bedside. The first-line pharmacotherapy is clonazapem 0.5–2 mg at bedtime. In addition, melatonin, donepezil, pramipexole and clonidine have been used in the treatment of RBD.

Nocturnal epilepsy can present with unusual night-time events. Approxi-mately 20% of patients with epilepsy have seizures exclusively in sleep. Similar to NREM parasomnias, patients with epilepsy may have amnesia for the events, which can occur during any part of the night. The defining behavioral feature is stereotypical activity. In nocturnal frontal lobe epilepsy (NFLE), there can be many events in a single night, as opposed to the lower frequency of other nocturnal seizures. In the evaluation of patients with nocturnal seizures, history is of extreme importance. Witness descriptions including the duration, quality of movement (stereotyped, focal or generalized), presence of bowel or bladder incontinence and time of night is paramount. A complete general and neurological examination should be performed. An MRI of the brain is helpful to assess for structural abnormalities and a sleep-deprived EEG may be helpful to identify interictal discharges. In patients with a frequency of once per week or more, video-EEG or video-EEG/PSG can be helpful in determining the diagnosis. The goal of treatment for patients with nocturnal events is freedom from seizures. Patients should be started on regular-release antiepileptic medi-cations that attain higher effective blood levels at night. Patients should avoid sleep deprivation and excessive alcohol use, which can lower the seizure threshold.

Psychogenic events may occur in isolation. Behaviors can be complex and dangerous; however, the movements are not stereotypical and the frequency can be variable. Patients have no or variable memory of these episodes.

Psychogenic events can occur at any time of night, but the characteristic PSG finding is that patients often wake up prior to episodes. Historical features regarding psychiatric disorders, polysubstance abuse, sexual or physical abuse and an assessment of stress should be investigated. Many patients may require a multipronged approach of pharmacotherapy and psychotherapy to improve events.

When evaluating patients with nocturnal events, clinicians may find a sleep diary helpful in defining the frequency and behavioral characteristics. Further evaluation by video-PSG is indicated for individuals with potential for injury, atypical features or symptoms of other sleep disorders.

The key feature in our patient's history was the stereotypical characteristic of the events. The similarity of behavior in each episode is a hallmark for epileptic seizures. The historical notation of witnessed events in the first half of the night is not uncommon in nocturnal seizures, especially as this is a time period when independent witnesses are more alert. The patient's wife typically did not go to sleep until 2.00 am, so her ability to recognize smaller events in the latter half of the night may have been diminished. The patient was initially labeled by his primary care physician as having sleep terrors based on the initial vocalization and lack of memory. Although possible, sleep terrors typically do not start in middle age. This case demonstrates how vocalization may occur at the start of a nocturnal seizure. Similarly, the episodes of fighting and punching the headboard would be reminiscent of RBD. Yet the patient did not have dream recall and his events did not vary in behavior. Stress was noted as a potential factor and a psychogenic mechanism was considered. The hallmark of psychogenic nocturnal events is their occurrence out of wakefulness. As a diagnosis of exclusion, this may be difficult to determine without PSG recording.

This patient had a normal sleep-deprived EEG; normal EEG activity in wakefulness is a common finding in patients with nocturnal epilepsy. Abnormalities may only be present in sleep. As Mr J. did not obtain sleep, the likelihood of seeing an interictal discharge was diminished. Given the patient's frequency of events, video-EEG monitoring was possible. Alternatively, a patient could have a PSG study with a full EEG electrode complement. Expansion of the EEG recording is necessary for the detection of focal seizures, as many of these may be isolated to areas that the limited EEG in PSG may not cover. For events of much lower frequency, a video-PSG with full EEG recording would have provided some information regarding the presence of interictal discharges and other potential sleep disorders (such as OSA). When studies show no disorder, a therapeutic trial with antiepileptic medication may be considered.

Pearls and gold

Nearly 3% of adults and 15% of children have nocturnal events.

Important questions to ask include level of consciousness, duration of the episode, time of the event, frequency of events, memory or dream recall, associated motor behaviors and stereotypy of motor behaviors.

Expansion of the nocturnal EEG recording is necessary for the detection of focal seizures, as many of these may be isolated to areas that the limited EEG in PSG may not cover.

Regular-release antiepileptic medications should be administered to attain higher effective blood levels at night.

Patients should avoid sleep deprivation and excessive alcohol use, which lower the seizure threshold.

SUGGESTED READING

HISTORICAL

Tinuper P, Cerullo A, Cirignotta F, *et al.* Nocturnal paroxysmal dystonia with short lasting attacks: three cases with evidence for an epileptic frontal lobe origin of seizures. *Epilepsia* 1990; **31**: 549–56.

REVIEWS

Mahowald M, Schenck C. Non-rapid eye movement sleep parasomnias. *Neurolog Clin* 2005; **23**: 1077–106.

Zucconi M, Ferini-Strambi L. NREM parasomnias: arousal disorders and differentiation from nocturnal frontal lobe epilepsy. *Clin Neurophysiol* 2000; **111** (Suppl. 2); S129–S35.

GENERAL

AASM (American Academy of Sleep Medicine). *International Classification of Sleep Disorders*, 2nd edn.: *Diagnostic and Coding Manual.* Westchester, Illinois: American Academy of Sleep Medicine, 2005.

Harris M, Grunstein R. Treatments for somnambulism in adults: assessing the evidence. *Sleep Med Rev* 2009; **13**: 295–7.

Pilon M, Montplaisir J, Zadra A. Precipitating factors of somnambulism: impact of sleep deprivation and forced arousals. *Neurology* 2008; **70**; 2274–5.

Plante DT, Winkelman J. Parasomnias. *Psychiatr Clin North Am* 2006; **29**: 969–87.

Posthuma RB, Gagnon JF, Vendette M, *et al.* Quantifying the risk of neurodegenerative disease in idiopathic REM sleep behavior disorder. *Neurology* 2009; **72**: 1296–300.

Part VI

Sleep and stroke

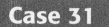

Sleep and stroke

Teresa Canet

Clinical history and examination

A 66-year-old man was found unresponsive in his house. On admission to hospital, he was normotensive with a Glasgow Coma Scale score of 5. He was intubated. Physical examination showed a fixed left pupil (right pupil was not assessable because of previous retinal detachment in that eye) and a Babinski response bilaterally. He had a history of hypertension, diabetes mellitus, stroke in the past with dysarthria and residual of facial paralysis. A CT scan of the head in the acute phase showed an old hypodense lesion in the right centrum semiovale. Twenty-four hours later, he was responsive to occasional verbal stimuli, showed severe hypersomnolence, vertical gaze palsy and mild left hemiparesis. A head CT 48 hours after hospitalization showed symmetric bilateral paramedian thalamic lesions suggestive of ischemia (Figure 31.1). He had episodes of cardiac asystole and ventricular tachycardia. An echocardiogram performed to rule out the presence of an intra-atrial thrombus showed a pattern of hypertensive heart disease with left ventricular concentric hypertrophy with good systolic function. Magnetic resonance angiography of the aortic arch demonstrated significant focal stenosis at the start of the initial segment of the right subclavian artery and a dominant left vertebral artery with diffuse atherosclerotic changes in the right vertebral artery. He required permanent cardiac pacing and anticoagulation therapy. During the first weeks of evolution, the patient had episodes of sudden worsening of his neurological status similar to a comatose state, but with regular breathing.

Special studies

A long-recording polysomnogram was registered to evaluate episodes of neurological impairment in the context of secondary hypersomnolence and acute

Case Studies in Sleep Neurology: Common and Uncommon Presentations, ed. A. Culebras. Published by Cambridge University Press. © Cambridge University Press 2010.

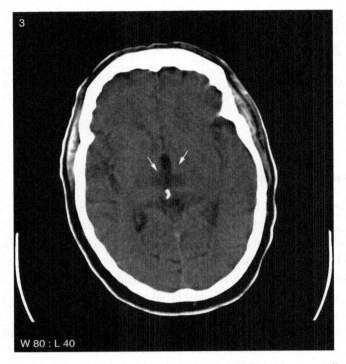

Figure 31.1 A CT scan of the head showing symmetric bilateral paramedian thalamic lesions.

bilateral paramedian thalamic infarctions. Several additional channels of EEG were added to investigate epileptiform activity.

Question

What is your diagnosis: seizures or pathological sleep?

Follow-up and results of studies

Polysomnography (PSG) recorded on the 15th day following the acute episode registered 17 hours (Figure 31.2) of brain activity. Total sleep time (TST) was 691 min (11.5 hours) and total wake time was 330 min (5.5 hours). Waking periods lasted about an hour. REM sleep time was 68 minutes, NREM sleep time was 623 minutes and slow-wave sleep time was 293 minutes (42% of TST). A short latency to stages N1, N2 and N3 was recorded. REM-sleep latency was 202 min. Sleep spindles were not identified. At 9.30pm, the patient became suddenly unresponsive following full wakefulness (Figure 31.3a), and the EEG revealed a pattern of stage N2 sleep (Figure 31.3b). Paroxystic activity was not observed.

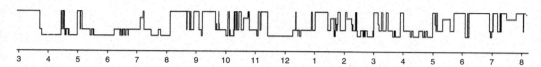

Figure 31.2 Hypnogram showing 17 hours of polysomnographic recording (from 3 pm to 8 am).

(a)

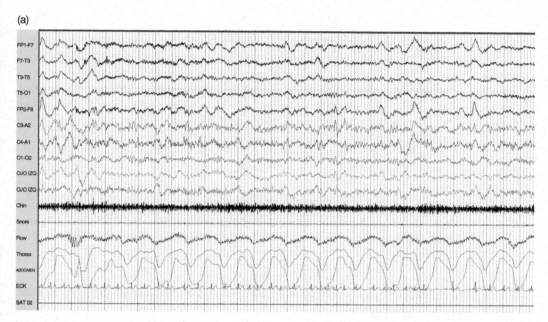

Figure 31.3a The awake EEG shows alpha and theta frequencies and muscle artifact. The figure represents a 30-second epoch. Sensitivity, 7 μV/mm, high-frequency filter, 15 cycles/s, low-frequency filter, 0.53 cycles/s.

Diagnosis

The diagnosis was hypersomnia with paroxysmal sleep associated with acute bilateral paramedian thalamic infarction, classified as hypersomnia of central origin (ICSD-2; AASM, 2005).

General remarks

The thalamus functions as a relay station in which sensory pathways coming from the spinal cord and brainstem form synapses on their way to the cerebral cortex. The thalamus has numerous connections with other areas of the brain as well, and these are thought to be important in the integration of cerebral, cerebellar

(b)

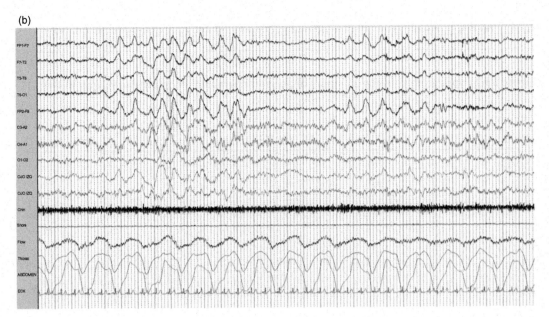

Figure 31.3b The stage N2 EEG shows theta frequency and K-complexes characterized by delta waves. Sleep spindles were not registered. The figure represents a 30-second epoch. Sensitivity, 7 μV/mm, high-frequency filter, 15 cycles/s, low-frequency filter, 0.53 cycles/s.

and brainstem activity. Thalamic infarctions result in markedly different clinical syndromes on the basis of their location.

Paramedian thalamic infarctions are associated with supranuclear palsy, somnolence, neuropsychological deficits and memory impairment. The clinical picture of this patient was typical. There was initial loss of consciousness followed by a hypersomnolent state in which sleep needs were markedly increased and the patient's ability to maintain attention was reduced. He presented the typical vertical gaze palsy and a mild motor deficit, without other oculomotor deficits, Horner's syndrome, dysarthria, gait ataxia, or mild sensory deficits or disorders of smell, taste and appetite. With improvement of consciousness, memory deficits became more evident. Paroxysmal sleep was another presenting symptom of this picture in the first weeks following the stroke. Bilateral thalamic infarcts may lead to more severe impairment of consciousness, a long-term recovery and an unfavorable outcome.

The infarction in this patient was in the territory of the paramedian thalamo-mesencephalic arteries. The medial aspects of the thalami and midbrain are supplied by the posterior circulation (vertebro-basilar system) via branches arising from proximal segments (P1) of the posterior cerebral arteries, called the mesencephalic arteries by José Segarra, a Spanish neuropathologist working in Boston in the 1960s (Segarra, 1970). In the same decade, Percheron, working in Paris, described three possible variations involving this arterial supply: small branches arising from both P1 segments, an asymmetrical common trunk arising from one of the P1 segments providing bilateral distribution (variation called the artery of Percheron) or an arterial arcade emanating from an artery bridging the two P1 segments (Percheron, 1977).

Bilateral thalamic infarcts are uncommon. When they happen, the paramedian thalamic regions are the most commonly affected. The infarcts are asymmetrical and caused by multiple emboli or small artery disease. Bilateral medial thalamic and rostral mesencephalic infarctions with a relatively symmetrical distribution should be recognized as due to occlusion of a possible single rare artery that is a normal variant: the artery of Percheron. The differential diagnosis includes the "top of the basilar artery" syndrome, where infarctions tend also to involve the territories supplied by the superior cerebellar and posterior cerebral arteries, and the occlusion of multiple vascular territories or other pathological conditions such as vasculitis or infectious disease.

Pearls and gold

Bilateral paramedian thalamic infarctions are unusual and are characterized by supranuclear palsy, hypersomnolence, neuropsychological deficits and memory impairment.

When bilateral medial thalamic infarctions are found in the context of hypersomnolence, occlusion of the artery of Percheron should be considered as the main diagnosis.

Performing conventional angiography may not be revealing, because lack of visualization of the artery does not exclude the presence of an occluded artery.

SUGGESTED READING

HISTORICAL

Percheron G. Les artères du thalamus humain: les artères choroïdiennes. *Rev Neurol (Paris)* 1977; **133**: 547–58.

Segarra JM. Cerebral vascular disease and behavior. I. The syndrome of the mesencephalic artery (basilar artery bifurcation). *Arch Neurol* 1970; **22**: 408–18.

REVIEW

Hermann DM, Siccoli M, Brugger P, *et al*. Evolution of neurological, neuropsychological and sleep-wake disturbances after paramedian thalamic stroke. *Stroke* 2008; **39**: 62–8.

GENERAL

AASM (American Academy of Sleep Medicine). *International Classification of Sleep Disorders*, 2nd edn.: *Diagnostic and Coding Manual*. Westchester, Illinois: American Academy of Sleep Medicine, 2005.

Bjornstad B, Goodman SH, Sirven JI, Dodick DW. Paroxysmal sleep as a presenting symptom of bilateral paramedian thalamic infarctions. *Mayo Clin Proc* 2003; **78**: 347–9.

Culebras A. Neuroanatomic and neurologic correlates of sleep disturbances. *Neurology* 1992; **42** (Suppl. 6): S19–S27.

Matheus MG, Castillo M. Imaging of acute bilateral paramedian thalamic and mesencephalic infarcts. *Am J Neuroradiol* 2003; **24**: 2005–8.

Rangel-Castilla L, Gasco J, Thompson B, Salinas P. Bilateral paramedian thalamic and mesencephalic infarcts after basilar tip aneurysm coiling: role of the artery of Percheron. *Neurochirurgia (Astur)* 2009; **20**: 288–93.

Part VII

Sleep-related movement disorders

Case 32

Violent tongue biting recurring during sleep

Roberto Vetrugno and Pasquale Montagna

Clinical history

A 60-year-old man was referred with a history of repeated episodes of painful tongue biting during sleep and finding it difficult to fall asleep because of racing thoughts and anxiety over whether he would be able to sleep on a given night. The first episode occurred at 56 years of age when one night the patient suddenly woke up feeling tongue pain. He was frightened when he saw blood-tinged saliva drooling out of his mouth, but soon realizing he had cut his tongue. Such episodes then occurred almost every night and at times several times during the same night, the patient often finding a blood-stained pillow upon rising in the morning and experiencing a sore tongue and teeth. Electroencephalograms showed slowing on left central derivations that was judged abnormal by referring physicians, although no spell was observed. Thereafter, carbamazepine (400 mg) was started with no effect on nocturnal tongue biting. The patient denied any history of bruxism or other sleep-related problems, and episodes of nocturnal tongue biting were never associated with limb jerking or incontinence or accompanied by transient loss of consciousness. The family history was negative for epilepsy, sleep disorders or any other significant neurological illness. According to his wife, as soon as the patient fell asleep, his teeth would start clicking throughout the night with a shaking sound.

Examination

Neurological examination was normal. In particular, chin tremor, oromandibular abnormal movements and masseter hypertrophy and tenderness on digital palpations were absent, and the temporomandibular joints were normal. No tooth wear was observed. A brain MRI was normal.

Laboratory parameters including serum chemistry (complete blood count, creatinine, electrolytes, liver enzymes, bilirubin, uric acid, lactate dehydrogenase, glucose, iron, ferritin, thyroid function) and neuropsychological examinations were normal.

Case Studies in Sleep Neurology: Common and Uncommon Presentations, ed. A. Culebras. Published by Cambridge University Press. © Cambridge University Press 2010.

Special studies and results

Brainstem acoustic evoked potentials, transcranial magnetic motor evoked potentials, blink reflex, facial and accessory nerve electroneurography, and electromyography of masseter, temporalis, mentalis and sternocleidomastoideus muscles were normal bilaterally. A wake EEG (using the International 10–20 system) did not show any paroxysmal activity and no motor events were elicited in wakefulness by acoustic startle stimulation or by electrical and tapping stimulations of the body, including the face on the forehead and glabella and the sternum.

All-night video-polysomnography (PSG) included EEG, right and left electrooculography, surface EMG of mentalis, masseter, orbicularis oculi, orbicularis oris, sternocleidomastoideus, deltoideus, rectus abdomins and tibialis anterior muscles, ECG, thoracic respirogram (by means of strain gauges placed at the level of the axilla), microphone (taped on the anterolateral part of the neck) and O_2 saturation (pulse oxymeter). Data were acquired on a Grass polygraph with a paper speed of 10 mm/s (30-second epochs) and synchronized video recording. EEG/EMG signals were filtered using a bandpass of 0.1–60 and 50–3,000 Hz respectively, and digitalized at a sampling rate of 1,024 Hz (Neuroscal Herdon), for subsequent offline analysis in 30-second epochs. Sleep data were staged according to standard international criteria, and sleep structure and sleep efficiency were evaluated. Transient arousals were scored as visible EEG arousals (usually alpha rhythm) lasting 2 seconds or longer and not associated with any stage/state change in the epoch scoring, with or without any body movements or respiratory event, and the arousal index (number of arousals per hour of sleep) was calculated. NREM sleep was also scored manually for the cyclic alternating pattern (CAP) sequences, defined as three or more A phases, i.e. transient complexes separated from each other by at least 2 and no more than 60 seconds of phase B (i.e. tonic theta/delta activities) and with the last A phase needed to end the sequence but not included in it. The CAP rate (percentage of NREM sleep occupied by CAP sequences) was then obtained.

Video-PSG recordings showed significantly decreased sleep efficiency (48%; normal value ≥85%), with total sleep time (TST) of 191 minutes (10% stage N1, 46% stage N2, 32% stage N3, 12% REM sleep) and wakefulness after sleep onset of 166 minutes. Sleep time with snoring (arbitrarily defined as the number of epochs with at least 50% of respiratory movements associated with snoring) amounted to 66 minutes (34% of TST) never associated with O_2 saturation below 92%. The mean arousal index was 23 (normal value <10) and the CAP rate during NREM sleep was 39% (35.9 ± 8.9% is the value reported in the literature for normal adulthood subjects).

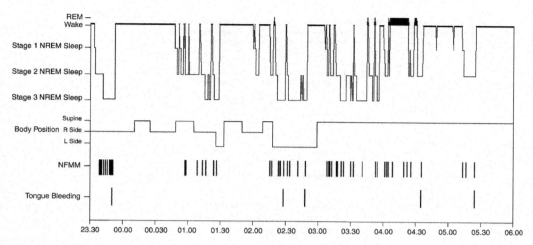

Figure 32.1 Sleep histogram showing recurrent nocturnal faciomandibular myoclonus (NFMM) complicated, in five episodes, with painful tongue bleeding.

During sleep, the patient had repeated episodes of sudden and forceful jaw closing with intense bite, corresponding to myoclonic EMG activity restricted to the temporalis, masseter, orbicularis oris and oculi muscles, and sometimes also involving the sternocleidomastoideus muscle. The EMG bursts recurred isolated or in clusters with two to four consecutive jerks, each lasting 50–150 ms and 100–500 μV in amplitude, and were often associated with tooth tapping sounds. The total number of episodes amounted to 53 with an index (number of episodes per hour of sleep) of 17. These appeared mainly during NREM sleep (47 episodes: 22 during stage N2 and 25 during stage N3) and occasionally during REM sleep (six episodes), but not as part of an overall and abnormal increased phasic muscle activity, and 38% were associated with sleep arousals (Figures 32.1 and 32.2). There was no relationship between snoring and the myoclonic activity, but CAP fluctuations seemed to influence the motor phenomena that appeared linked to CAP phase A in 68% of cases. On five occasions, the sudden intense bites woke the patient up due to painful tongue lacerations with bleeding located on the tip (Figure 32.2). None of the sleep EEG recordings displayed any epileptiform activity. Grinding and gnashing sounds with phasic (duration 0.25–2 seconds), tonic (>2 seconds) or mixed (tonic activity interspaced with more phasic muscle activation) masticatory EMG activity, typical of sleep bruxism, were never observed.

EMG analysis of the myoclonic bursts showed that the first activated muscles were always the masseter and the temporalis, followed by the orbicularis oris and oculi after a variable delay of 10–20 ms and, when present, by the sternocleidomastoideus after a delay of 25–30 ms.

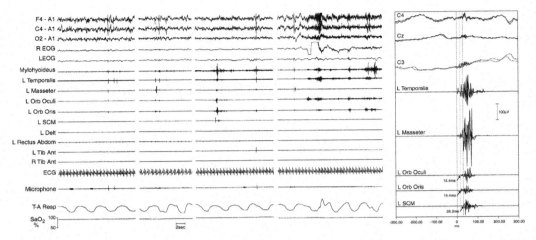

Figure 32.2 Polysomnographic recording showing multiple episodes of myoclonic jerks involving the orofacial, masticatory and (in one episode) the cervical sternocleidomastoideus (SCM) muscles during NREM sleep. In the last episodes, the patient suddenly woke up following the bite that caused painful laceration on the tip portion of the tongue with bleeding. Back-averaging of EEG activity related to the myoclonic jerks (right panel; two series: 20 consecutive faciomandibular jerks each) triggered on the masseter muscle and showing EMG activity starting in the temporalis-masseter followed by orbicularis oculi-oris and then SCM activity with a mean delay of 15.4 and 28.2 ms, without any preceding jerk-related cortical EEG potential. EOG, electro-oculogram; Orb Oculi, orbicularis oculi; Orb Oris, orbicularis oris; SCM, sternocleidomastoideus; Delt, deltoideus; Rectus Abd, rectus abdominis; Tib Ant, tibialis anterior; ECG, electrocardiogram; T-A Resp, thoraco-abdominal respirogram; SaO_2, O_2 saturation; R, right; L, left.

Back-averaging of EEG activity related to the myoclonic bursts, performed by averaging 20 consecutive jerks, did not show any jerk-related cortical EEG potential and confirmed that the masseter and temporalis EMG preceded both the orbicularis oculi and orbicularis oris with a mean delay of 15.4 ms and subsequently the sternocleidomastoideus with a mean delay of 28.2 ms (Figure 32.2).

Thereafter, treatment with carbamazepine was stopped and substituted with clonazepam 1 mg daily, which resulted in the patient becoming symptom-free. Currently, the patient has been on clonazepam for more than 12 months and the nocturnal tongue biting has never recurred.

Question

Does the patient have seizures or myoclonic jerks?

Follow-up

The PSG recording of the patient described here revealed that he suffered from nocturnal myoclonic jerks involving the masseter and orbicularis oculi and oris muscles, sometimes also spreading to the sternocleidomastoideus, and leading to troublesome tongue biting and bleeding during sleep with subsequent disordered sleep. Sleep-induced faciomandibular myoclonus in our patient recurred mainly during NREM sleep and seemed to have a subcortical origin. Indeed, there was no jerk-related EEG preceding activity and the EEG/EMG back-averaging analysis suggested that it originated in a circuitry from V–VII-innervated muscles along a polysynaptic pathway, with possible volley until the XI innervated muscle(s), in some respects resembling brainstem reticular myoclonus. However, at variance from reticular myoclonus, myoclonic activity could not be evoked in a reflex way in our patient and remained restricted to sleep.

Diagnosis

The diagnosis was nocturnal faciomandibular myoclonus.

Nocturnal faciomandibular myoclonus should be differentiated from epileptic myoclonus and from extrapyramidal involuntary movements during sleep. Although clinical seizure activity may have no scalp EEG correlates, the presence of the tongue bite at the tip, the absence of epileptiform EEG activity on back-averaging and the lack of response to carbamazepine make an epileptic patho-genesis of sleep-induced myoclonic tongue biting unlikely. Extrapyramidal involuntary movements are generally considered to disappear during sleep. Nonetheless, non-rhythmic movement disorders have been described to be acti-vated during sleep in patients with evident brainstem lesions, although they involve mainly the arms, legs and thighs, appear also during daytime wakefulness and are composed of tonic and tonic–phasic contractions, which is different from the sleep-related faciomandibular myoclonus recorded in this patient. Other conditions in which tongue biting during sleep may be observed, i.e. rhythmic movement disorders and hereditary chin trembling, were excluded either by clinical examination or PSG.

General remarks

The relationship between sleep-related faciomandibular myoclonus and sleep bruxism should be addressed. Patients are defined as sleep bruxers when they present with more than four phasic (0.25–2 seconds), tonic (>2 seconds) or mixed (phasic–tonic) bruxism episodes per hour of sleep, with an EMG ampli-tude of at least 20% of the maximum voluntary contraction; or more than

25 bruxism bursts per hour of sleep and at least one episode with a grinding sound per sleep period. Tooth wear is frequent in bruxers and the continuous lateral movement of the jaw results in temporomandibular joint dysfunction like disk displacement. Rhythmic, phasic, tonic or mixed jaw muscle EMG activity typical of bruxism was absent in our patient, and a lateral or protrusive/retrusive jaw position was not observed. The jaw movements were instead myoclonic and vertical and could also involve the cervical muscles.

Further studies are needed to understand the source and the natural course of this sleep disorder. Although nocturnal faciomandibular myoclonus is classified under sleep bruxism in the present ICSD-2 (AASM, 2005), it should be kept distinct from bruxism and other epileptic and non-epileptic movement disorders during sleep. Our case emphasizes the need to check patients' sleep-related spells by means of video-PSG and detailed neurophysiological studies for a complete characterization with the aim of avoiding delays before establishing the correct diagnosis and promptly instituting the appropriate treatment.

Pearls and gold

In faciomandibular myoclonus, the jaw movements are myoclonic and vertical and may involve the cervical muscles.

The presence of a tongue bite at the tip, the absence of epileptiform EEG activity on back-averaging and the lack of response to carbamazepine make an epileptic pathogenesis of sleep-induced myoclonic tongue biting unlikely.

SUGGESTED READING

HISTORICAL

Aguglia U, Gambardella A, Quattrone A. Sleep-induced masticatory myoclonus: a rare parasomnia associated with insomnia. *Sleep* 1991; **14**: 80–2.

REVIEW

Loi D, Provini F, Vetrugno R, *et al.* Sleep-related faciomandibular myoclonus: a sleep-related movement disorder different from bruxism. *Mov Disord* 2007; **22**: 1819–22.

GENERAL

AASM (American Academy of Sleep Medicine). *International Classification of Sleep Disorders*, 2nd edn.: *Diagnostic and Coding Manual*. Westchester, Illinois: American Academy of Sleep Medicine, 2005.

Lavigne GJ, Manzini C, Kato T. Sleep bruxism. In: Kryger M, Roth T, Dement W, eds. *Principles and Practice of Sleep Medicine*, 4th edn. Philadelphia: WB Saunders Co., 2005; 946–59.

Vasiknanonte P, Kuasirikul S, Vasiknanonte S. Two faces of nocturnal tongue biting. *J Med Assoc Thail* 1997; **80**: 500–7.

Vetrugno R, Provini F, Plazzi G, *et al.* Familial nocturnal facio-mandibular myoclonus mimicking sleep bruxism. *Neurology* 2002; **58**: 644–7.

A child with behavioral problems and violent sleep behavior leading to trauma

Mark Eric Dyken and Deborah C. Lin-Dyken

Clinical history

A girl of 8 years and 5 months with a history of attention deficit hyperactivity disorder (ADHD) was admitted to address significant behavioral problems that included prolonged rocking behaviors that often disrupted the patient's sleep. A comprehensive medical and behavioral evaluation with sleep monitoring was planned to develop a focused management plan.

The patient's mother reported that her daughter's bedtime ranged from 8 to 8.30 pm, with a waking time of 6.30 am. Her sleep latency was described as being prolonged, with frequent arousals once sleep was attained, during which she might get up and "run around" in the middle of the night. The patient was frequently found in bed humming and rocking, during which time she objectively appeared to be either awake or asleep. These behaviors were similar to the rocking and humming she would demonstrate when upset during the day. Although the patient had a history of temper tantrums, her behavior had improved over the previous 2 years. Nevertheless, she had persistent episodes of nocturnal rocking. She had fallen out of bed on several occasions, after which violent body movements continued while lying on the hard floor surface, often leading to blunt head trauma with epistaxis.

The patient was the full-term product of a normal vaginal delivery, of a mother who denied the use of cigarettes, alcohol, illicit drugs or any medications during the pregnancy. There were previous reports of child maltreatment (denial of critical care) related to the patient's failure to thrive, which was diagnosed at 2.5 months. After that time, she attained her developmental milestones appropriately until she entered kindergarten, at which time her teachers felt that her behavior warranted an assessment for ADHD and necessitated that she repeat kindergarten. At admission, she was in the second grade in a multi-categorical classroom with some limited integration. There were no past surgeries, injuries or significant illnesses other than chickenpox; her immunizations were up to date

Case Studies in Sleep Neurology: Common and Uncommon Presentations, ed. A. Culebras. Published by Cambridge University Press. © Cambridge University Press 2010.

and no allergies were reported. Her only medication was methylphenidate 15 mg q 7 am, and 5 mg at noon and at 3.30 pm.

The family history was positive for ADHD and behavioral problems in her brother, who continued to have enuresis at the age of 6 years and also had similar rocking behaviors when upset. It was noted that the behavior of these siblings tended to worsen significantly when they were in the presence of each other. The patient also had maternal uncles with behavioral problems and a maternal grandmother with bipolar affective disorder, and there were reports of paternal alcohol abuse. The review of systems was positive for enuresis twice a week (nightly until 6.5 years).

Examination

Vital signs were unremarkable, and developmentally she was Tanner stage 1, with a weight of 27.4 kg (75th percentile) and a height of 130.5 cm (25th percentile). A formal evaluation by a dentist indicated that the patient had a healthy mouth. The general examination showed small injuries on the left forearm, with scabbed-over injuries on the left lower leg and right upper arm. Neurologically, she was noted to have tight heel cords with mild right foot weakness, diffusely brisk muscle stretch reflexes, with 4–5 beats of right ankle clonus and 2–3 beats of left ankle clonus.

Question

Is the patient having seizures or suffering from a motor disorder of sleep?

Special studies and results

Complete blood count, serum lead, free erythrocyte protoporphyrins, urine analysis and tuberculin skin tests were unremarkable. An MRI of the brain was performed to rule out neurological injury given the tight heel cords, brisk muscle stretch reflexes and right foot weakness. It was of note that the patient could not tolerate the study and required sedation, which could not be attained using chloral hydrate, and general anesthesia was necessary. This imaging study was normal.

A cognitive evaluation using selected subtests from the Wechsler Intelligence Scale for Children – Revised was performed. Her lowest scores were in verbal abilities; the Preschool Language Scale 3 indicated an auditory comprehension level at 6 years, 1 month, and an expressive communication level at 6 years,

5 months. The overall impression of this testing was low average intellectual functioning.

The Bruininks–Oseretsky Test of Motor Proficiency showed gross overall motor skills at approximately the 6 year, 9 month level; visual motor control at approximately 5 years, 8 months; upper limb speed and dexterity at approximately 6 years, 8 months. The Visual Motor Integration Test scored at approximately 5 years, 10 months age equivalent, and the Motor Free Visual Perception Test scored at approximately 6 years, 8 months age equivalency. During one evaluation, she stood at the table and began to rock back and forth from foot to foot, but continued to participate quite well in the testing process. The impression from this evaluation was a mild to moderate delay in fine motor and perceptual skills, commensurate with cognitive functioning.

Given the history of child maltreatment, the Structured Anatomical Doll Interview was performed. The results were similar to those of non-abused children, rather than those with documented histories of sexual abuse.

The patient underwent an extended four-phase functional analysis to assess her responsiveness to environment and medication variations. During a double-blind medication trial to test the effectiveness of her admission dose of methylphenidate, no significant differences were noted in her behavior off or on methylphenidate. In addition, differential reinforcement of appropriate behaviors (positively rewarding behaviors considered good, and avoiding frank punishments) reduced problematic behaviors almost completely.

Polysomnography (PSG) performed on the first night of admission with split-screen video monitoring was relatively unremarkable. Her sleep efficiency was 86.45%, with no evidence of apnea, hypopnea, significant O_2 desaturation, snoring, parasomnia or seizure-like activity. There were occasional myoclonic movements with no evidence of frank periodic limb movements of sleep (PLMS), with a movement index of 6.1 events per hour and a movement/arousal index of 2.0.

Following the initial PSG, simple videotaping was performed on each subsequent night during the hospitalization. During the first four nights, the patient's sleep was described as restless. Beginning with the fifth night, she began to exhibit five to six episodes of rocking per night. These events were reported as frequent apparent awakenings with body rocking and less frequently with head banging: "Lots of rocking behavior out of self-control, but manageable." During one episode, she suffered blunt trauma to the nose, with mild epistaxis that resolved readily. No frank correlations were recognized between her sleep patterns and daytime behavioral problems.

Given the recurrence of persistent nocturnal body movements documented with continuous, in-room video monitoring, a repeat PSG was performed with

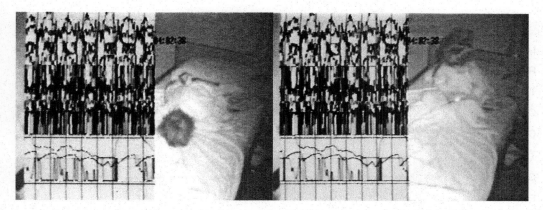

Figure 33.1 The pictures show an 8-year-old female during relatively violent nocturnal behavior, evidenced as head banging associated with very rhythmic 0.5–2 Hz anterior–posterior movements of the body. In this figure, a full movement cycle can be appreciated to occur within a 1-second period at 04:02:38 hours.

split-screen video monitoring. This study revealed five discrete episodes of head banging, body rocking and/or leg banging (Figure 33.1). The patient experienced 59 minutes of relatively violent body movements throughout the night. These episodes of movement would generally begin abruptly from stage N1 or N2 sleep and after ending were immediately followed by stage N1, stage N2 or REM sleep (Figure 33.2). Four of the events were strongly associated with K-complexes in N2 sleep. No epileptiform activity was appreciated.

Diagnosis

The diagnosis was sleep-related rhythmic movement disorder.

Follow-up

The patient's history and PSG analysis are classical for rhythmic movement disorder (RMD); classified in ICSD-2 (AASM, 2005) as a sleep-related movement disorder. Rhythmic movements of the body during drowsy wakefulness and sleep are common in normal infants and children, reportedly occurring in 59% of all infants at 9 months of age, in 33% of all children at 18 months and in 5% of the population by 5 years of age. As such, rhythmic movements in sleep and drowsiness can only be considered a disorder if they interfere significantly with sleep, impair daytime function or result in injury.

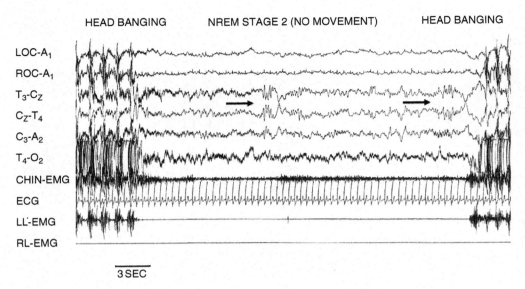

HEAD BANGING   NREM STAGE 2 (NO MOVEMENT)   HEAD BANGING

LOC-A$_1$
ROC-A$_1$
T$_3$-C$_z$
C$_z$-T$_4$
C$_3$-A$_2$
T$_4$-O$_2$
CHIN-EMG
ECG
LL-EMG
RL-EMG

3 SEC

Figure 33.2 Immediately after and preceding a prolonged period of typical head banging, the patient stops moving for an approximate 28-second period, at which time the EEG shows unequivocal stage N2 sleep with characteristic 12–14 Hz sleep spindles and K-complexes (indicated by the two black arrows) with well-defined negative sharp waves followed by a positive component. One K-complex immediately precedes the resumption of head banging. LOC, left outer canthus; ROC, right outer canthus; A1, left ear; T, temporal; C, central; O, occipital; ECG, electrocardiogram; LL, left leg; RL, right leg. (Modified with permission from Figure 1 in Dyken et al., 1997.)

Although one study found higher anxiety scores in children with body rocking than in controls, most patients with sleep-related rhythmic movements are otherwise normal. In older children and adults, there may be a higher association with intellectual disabilities (mental retardation) and autism. In the developmentally delayed, there have been reports of soft tissue injuries, with significant injury being rare.

The differential diagnosis for episodic self-injurious behaviors includes tantrums, self-abuse, seizures and parasomnias (such as sleepwalking, night terrors and REM-sleep behavior disorder). In addition, RMD-like behaviors have been reported to improve in a subject with restless legs syndrome (RLS) and sleep apnea after treatment with continuous positive airway pressure therapy (Gharagozlou et al., 2009).

In RMD, the subtypes of movement include body rocking, head banging and head rolling (and less commonly body rolling, leg banging or leg rolling), often in association with rhythmic humming or oral sounds that are otherwise inarticulate. The movement frequency is usually between 0.5 and 2.0 movements per second, whereas the duration of any given period of repetitive movement is generally less than 15 minutes.

Patients are amnestic for sleep-related rhythmic movements, whereas events during drowsiness generally can be recalled. One study of six children with RMD found that 3 weeks of controlled sleep restriction with the concomitant use of hypnotics during the first week of therapy led to an almost complete resolution of pathological movements. To the authors, this therapeutic success suggests that the RMD results from a voluntary self-soothing behavior.

Given reportedly higher anxiety scores in some children with body rocking, and the suggestion that in older children there may be a higher association with cognitive and adaptive disabilities (mental retardation), therapies were directed toward aggressively addressing presumed underlying psychosocial issues. At the end of the patient's hospitalization, her overall behavior was reported to be under good control after the modification of her environment.

In regard to cognitive disability, her learning deficits were aggressively addressed in the school setting, with recommendations that her language be monitored by the school's speech language pathologist, and that her primary teacher, after consultation with neuropsychologists, ensure appropriate language stimulation in the classroom.

To address the patient's mild gross motor delay, there was a recommendation for continued opportunities to engage in a variety of gross motor activities, with caution regarding those requiring balance or bilateral coordination. To address behavioral issues, methylphenidate was discontinued, and differential reinforcement of appropriate behavior was recommended in school and at home, and a maximum respite service was provided at home (to provide adequate, trained and specialized care for the two children with ADHD when the parents were not at home), with additional help in the classroom for up to a 6-month period. An ongoing video recording of the patient in her natural school environment to document progress was recommended.

The patient's family was dependent on state support with regard to medical care. Given the relatively violent nature of these events, the video analysis of the events was used successfully in court as evidence that justified the use of a hospital safety bed at home, equipped with side rails and padding in order to prevent any serious injury.

General remarks

Rhythmic movement disorder was initially formally classified as a sleep/wake transition parasomnia in the *International Classification of Sleep Disorders, Revised: Diagnostic and Coding Manual* (ASDA, 1997). At the time of this

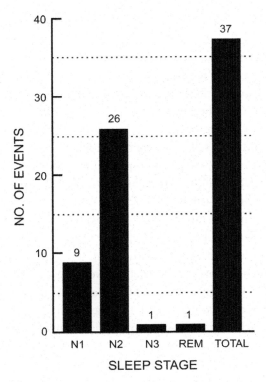

Figure 33.3 RMD is strongly associated with stage N2 sleep and K-complex activity. In this study, 26 events were associated with stage N2 sleep (20 with K-complex), one event was observed in stage N3 sleep and one occurred in REM sleep, while only nine total events appeared in stage N1 sleep. (Modified with permission from Figure 2, in Dyken *et al.*, 1997).

manual's publication, it was appreciated that, although RMD could also occur during full wakefulness and alertness (particularly in individuals with intellectual disabilities or mental retardation), when RMD was associated with sleep, it generally occurred during sleep onset or in the transition from wakefulness to sleep.

In 1997, a video-PSG study of children aged 1–12 years, referred for the evaluation of relatively violent nocturnal behaviors, characterized the movement, level of responsiveness and sleep stage during each patient's typical spell. Thirty-seven periods of head banging, body rocking and leg banging were strongly associated with sleep; 26 events were associated with stage N2 sleep (20 with K-complexes), one appeared in stage N3 sleep and one occurred in REM sleep, whereas only nine events were recognized in stage N1 sleep (Figure 33.3).

Given these findings, RMD could no longer be considered a phenomenon isolated only to simple drowsiness and the transition from wakefulness to sleep.

This issue was successfully addressed in ICSD-2 (AASM, 2005), as RMD has formally been reclassified as a sleep-related movement disorder rather than as a sleep/wake transition parasomnia.

Pearls and gold

Sleep-related RMD occurs in the transitions to sleep (stage N1), but is also strongly associated with stage N2 of sleep and less frequently with stage N3 and REM sleep.

Subtypes of movement include body rocking, head banging, head rolling and less commonly body rolling, leg banging or leg rolling, often in association with rhythmic humming or oral sounds that are otherwise inarticulate.

In older children, there may be a higher association of sleep-related RMD with intellectual disabilities (mental retardation).

SUGGESTED READING

REVIEW

Dyken ME, Lin-Dyken DC, Yamada T. Diagnosing rhythmic movement disorder with video-polysomnography. *Pediatr Neurol* 1997; **16**: 37–41.

GENERAL

AASM (American Academy of Sleep Medicine). *International Classification of Sleep Disorders, 2nd edn.: Diagnostic and Coding Manual.* Westchester, Illinois: American Academy of Sleep Medicine, 2005.

ASDA (American Sleep Disorders Association). *International Classification of Sleep Disorders, Revised: Diagnostic and Coding Manual.* Rochester, Minnesota: American Sleep Disorders Association, 1997.

Etzioni T, Katz N, Hering E, *et al.* Controlled sleep restriction for rhythmic movement disorder. *J Pediatr* 2005; **3**: 393–5.

Gharagozlou P, Seyffert M, Santos R, *et al.* Rhythmic movement disorder associated with respiratory arousals and improved by CPAP titration in a patient with restless legs syndrome and sleep apnea. *Sleep Med* 2009; **4**: 501–3.

Case 34

Clicking all night

Maha Alattar

Clinical history

Mrs. H. was a 45-year-old female homemaker who presented at the sleep clinic with symptoms of daytime fatigue, sleepiness and chronic headaches for the past 2 years. Her husband, who accompanied her, noticed that she made clicking sounds with her mouth "all night long." She woke up with severe headache and soreness of her jaw and face. This pain limited activities such as chewing and talking. During emotional distress, she clenched her jaw. She admitted to moderate depression and stress at home related to psychosocial issues with her teenage daughter.

She consumed one cup of caffeinated tea during the day, but no alcohol, tobacco or illicit drugs. She did not exercise. She maintained regular bed and wake-up times and tried to get 8 hours of sleep each night. However, her sleep was described as restless with frequent tossing. She did not report symptoms of restless legs, dream enactment or narcolepsy. Her medical health included hypertension and allergic rhinitis. She currently takes one antihypertensive medication.

Examination

The patient's vital signs were normal. Her BMI was elevated (34 kg/m^2). Mild nasal congestion was noted. The uvula was mildly congested and the oropharyngeal space was Mallampati score class 2–3. Bilateral masseter muscle hypertrophy was visible. A facial and oral examination revealed significant tenderness to palpation of the jaw muscles (masseter and lateral pterygoids) and the temporalis muscles. Jaw opening was very limited secondary to pain; temporomandibular clicking was elicited. Teeth wear was evident. Pain was elicited to digital palpation of lower dentition. The inner cheeks revealed teeth indentations. The neurological and general examinations were otherwise normal.

Case Studies in Sleep Neurology: Common and Uncommon Presentations, ed. A. Culebras. Published by Cambridge University Press. © Cambridge University Press 2010.

Special studies

Nocturnal polysomnography (PSG), a basic metabolic work-up and a thyroid function test were carried out.

Question

What is your diagnosis?

Results of studies

Polysomnographic recording showed frequent episodes of sleep bruxism in the EMG channel that occurred during NREM light sleep (Figure 34.1). The EMG leads showed repetitive bursting activity of the jaw muscle. Video and audio recordings confirmed teeth grinding episodes. In addition, snoring with related

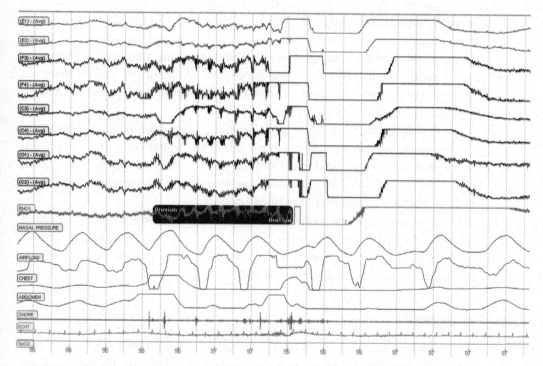

Figure 34.1 Electromyographic recording during routine PSG shows a series of ten phasic–rhythmic EMG activity bursts (nearly 1 per second) that are transmitted to the EEG and EOG leads. Jaw movement and tooth grinding were confirmed with video and audio recording.

arousals were noted, but without apneas or hypoxemia. Periodic limb movements of sleep (PLMS) were not identified. A basic metabolic panel and thyroid tests were normal.

Diagnosis

The principal diagnosis was bruxism (sleep and awake). Secondary diagnoses were primary snoring with arousals, chronic daily headache, daytime dysfunction with fatigue, sleepiness, depression, and obesity. Sleep-related bruxism is classified as a sleep-related movement disorder in ICSD-2 (AASM, 2005).

Follow-up

This case illustrates the complexity of symptoms in patients with bruxism such that they can be multiple and inter-related and therefore must be addressed with a comprehensive and multidisciplinary approach. The sleep specialist addressed the diagnoses, reviewed the results of the study and laboratory results, and provided education on bruxism, the related headaches and snoring, and discussed the causes of fatigue. The specialist proceeded with the appropriate management. The goal of treatment focused on a reduction of the frequency of bruxism, ameliorating facial pain/headaches, protection of dentition, improvement of daytime symptoms (fatigue, depression) and treatment of snoring and related arousals.

An oral appliance through a local pharmacy was recommended in lieu of a custom-made appliance as she could not afford the dental visits. Stress reduction techniques were emphasized and a heating pad was recommended to be applied to the jaw muscles in order to reduce muscle tension in the evening and at night-time. A muscle relaxant was prescribed.

Optimal sleep hygiene was emphasized. The patient was advised to begin a regimen of weight loss through exercise and healthy eating habits to improve her mood and fatigue and decrease the snoring. A corticosteroid nasal spray was prescribed to reduce the allergic rhinitis.

General remarks

The word bruxism stems from the Greek word *brychein*, which means "to gnash the teeth." Bruxism is defined as an involuntary and repetitive movement of the jaw muscles that causes grinding and/or clenching of the teeth. Jaw clenching in an awake and aware individual is termed awake bruxism. Sleep-related bruxism (SB), on the other hand, is noted by the bed partner and causes symptoms and signs such as morning headaches, jaw/facial pain and clicking and grinding sounds. Sleep-related bruxism has a prevalence of 8% in the general population. Bruxism is often diagnosed by routine dental visits and less frequently by a sleep specialist. Consequences of bruxism include temporomandibular disorders such as jaw pain and limitation of movement, chronic headaches, disrupted sleep of the patient and bed partner, and dental wear.

The pathophysiology of SB is under ongoing investigation. Recent studies suggest that sleep bruxism occurs at sleep-stage transitions, especially before REM sleep. Genetic and behavioral factors such as stress also play a role, but gender does not.

Electromyographic recordings during PSG reveal jaw muscle activity of three types: phasic (three or more bursts of muscle contractions at 1 Hz), which cause the rhythmic muscle activity; tonic (contraction that lasts >2 seconds), which causes sustained activity; and mixed. Sleep-related bruxism often occurs in NREM sleep, especially in the lighter stages of sleep. The PSG diagnostic cut-off criteria for SB have not been established; the following criteria were suggested by Huynh *et al.* (2006): (1) more than four bruxism episodes per hour; (2) more than six bruxism bursts per episode and/or 25 bruxism bursts per hour of sleep; and (3) at least two episodes with grinding sounds.

Studies have reported that SB occurs in association with primary sleep disorders such as obstructive sleep apnea (OSA). Treatment of the OSA with continuous positive airway pressure (CPAP) therapy or other modalities eliminated or nearly eradicated the tooth grinding events. Secondary bruxism may occur as a result of a neurological disorder (Parkinson's disease), a psychiatric disease (schizophrenia) or medication administration of selective serotonin reuptake inhibitors (SSRIs).

Treatment of SB needs to be case specific and should center on the prevention of the associated conditions (i.e. stress, dental malocclusion and sleep apnea) and is aimed at protecting the teeth and temporomandibular joints while improving the sleep quality. Management can be divided into dental, behavioral and pharmacological. Any other primary sleep disorders (as sleep apnea or PLMS) that might lead to EEG arousals and potentially to episodes of bruxism should be treated. It is prudent for any physician who treats patients with headaches to consider bruxism in the differential diagnosis.

Additional recommendations include consultation with a dentist or orthodontist to evaluate and treat a misaligned jaw or dental malocclusion. Intra-oral mouth guards or splints are often prescribed to protect dentition, but their effectiveness in treating SB is less clear. Custom-made splints are recommended. However, over-the-counter boil-and-bite mouth guards are available if the patient is unable to afford the custom-made mouth guards.

Behavioral modification should be part of the treatment plan and includes optimal sleep hygiene, stress reduction techniques such as yoga and guided imagery, and addressing and treating underlying mood disorders. Application of a warm washcloth or heating pad to the jaw area prior to bedtime to ease muscle tension may help. Avoiding foods, medications and habits that potentially worsen bruxism such as caffeine, alcohol, antipsychotic medications (unless required) and chewing gum is desirable.

Pharmacological intervention including muscle relaxants, benzodiazepines (clonazepam), catecholaminergic products (levodopa, clonidine), gabapentin and buspirone are reserved for severe cases. Botox injection in selected patients has been helpful.

Pearls and gold

Consequences of bruxism include temporomandibular joint pain with limitation of movement, chronic headaches, disrupted sleep of the patient and bed partner, and dental wear.

Management includes dental correction, behavioral counseling and pharmacological intervention.

SUGGESTED READING

REVIEWS

Koyano K, Tsukiyama Y, Ichiki R, Kuwata. Assessment of bruxism in the clinic. *J Oral Rehabil* 2008; **35**: 495–508.
Lavigne GJ, Khoury S, Abe S, Yamaguchi T, Raphael K. Bruxism physiology and pathology: an overview for clinicians. *J Oral Rehabil* 2008; **35**: 476–94.

GENERAL

AASM (American Academy of Sleep Medicine). *International Classification of Sleep Disorders*, 2nd edn.: *Diagnostic and Coding Manual*. Westchester, Illinois: American Academy of Sleep Medicine, 2005.
Huynh N, Lavigne GJ, Lanfranchi PA, Montplaisir JY, de Champlain J. The effect of 2 sympatholytic medications – propranolol and clonidine – on sleep bruxism: experimental randomized controlled studies. *Sleep* 2006; **29**: 307–16.
Lavigne GJ, Rompré PH, Montplaisir JY. Sleep bruxism: validity of clinical research diagnostic criteria in a controlled polysomnographic study. *J Dent Res* 1996; **75**: 546–52.

Macedo CR, Silva AB, Machado MA, Saconato H, Prado GF. Occlusal splints for treating sleep bruxism (tooth grinding). *Cochrane Database Syst Rev* 2007; **17**: CD005514.

Oksenberg A, Arons E. Sleep bruxism related to obstructive sleep apnea: the effect of continuous positive airway pressure. *Sleep Med* 2002; **3**: 513–5.

Schwartz M, Freund B. Treatment of temporomandibular disorders with botulinum toxin. *Clin J Pain* 2002; **18** (6 Suppl.): S198–S203.

Repetitive arm movements

Maha Alattar and Bradley V. Vaughn

Clinical history

Mr. D. was a 48-year-old right-handed man whose chief complaints were heavy snoring, witnessed apneas, frequent awakenings at night and daytime fatigue with sleepiness. His bedtime was 10 pm; he fell asleep quickly and got out of bed at 5 am. In the morning he felt refreshed; however, he needed coffee to retain his daytime energy. He drank about 6–12 cups of coffee in the morning/afternoon and his Epworth Sleepiness Scale score was 8 (see Appendix). His wife mentioned that he "moved his arms and legs a lot at night" such that it made it difficult for her to share the bed with him. The patient did not recount symptoms of restless legs syndrome (RLS), hypnagogic hallucinations, sleep paralysis or cataplexy. He denied complex behaviors such as yelling, speaking, rocking or other rhythmic movements. He complained of a 4-year history of neck pain and right shoulder pain with spasms that radiated down his right arm and elbow with some morning stiffness. Mr. D. denied weakness, numbness or tingling in his extremities. The patient worked in a processing plant and part of his duties involved repetitive arm movements. He denied the use of tobacco, alcohol or recreational drugs.

His medical history included cluster headaches, mild depression and right rotator cuff damage. His medications included citalopram and an acetaminophen hydrocodone combination for shoulder pain.

Examination

Vital signs were normal and his BMI was 28 kg/m^2. A nasal examination revealed mild nasal congestion and an oral examination showed a Mallampati score of class 3. The general examination was otherwise normal except for pain on movement of the right shoulder and arm. A neck examination showed good

Case Studies in Sleep Neurology: Common and Uncommon Presentations, ed. A. Culebras. Published by Cambridge University Press. © Cambridge University Press 2010.

mobility with a full range of motion. Paravertebral muscle spasm was not present. An examination of the extremities revealed a normal range of motion of all joints. No joint swelling/erythema was noted.

A neurological examination was normal with the exception of sensory deficit to pin prick and light touch in the forearm, thumb and index finger on the right side; his reflexes were slightly depressed in the right arm.

Special studies

Nocturnal polysomnography (PSG), a basic metabolic work-up, and B12, folate and thyroid function tests were carried out.

Question

What is your diagnosis?

Results of studies

Polysomnographic recordings confirmed the following:

1. Diagnostic PSG: obstructive sleep apnea–hypopnea syndrome (OSAHS) with an apnea–hypopnea index (AHI) of 9 events per hour; supine AHI was 17 events per hour.
2. Polysomnography of the arm and leg surface EMG activity was recorded during both studies (diagnostic and continuous positive airway pressure [CPAP]). Stereotypical periodic movements were seen on video recording that also showed periodic dorsiflexion of both feet and flexion of the arms. The diagnostic PSG showed 505 periodic limb movements of sleep (PLMS) with a periodic limb movement (PLM) index of 66 per hour; 392 were associated with arousals with a resulting PLM arousal index of 52 per hour. During CPAP titration, there were 500 PLMS with an index of 80 per hour; the PLM arousal index was 72.

An interesting pattern was noted in the diagnostic and CPAP studies. Periodic arm movements of sleep (PAMS) were a significant part of the patient's PLMs. Periodic arm movements dominated the first third of the night, whereas periodic leg movements dominated the latter third of the night. The middle third included a mixed picture of arm and leg movements. All movements were clearly viewed on video.

A basic metabolic panel, B12 and thyroid tests were normal. His ferritin level was 48. An MRI of the cervical spine showed multilevel degenerative changes with a small bulging disc at C6–C7 with moderate bilateral neural foraminal stenosis at that level, but no nerve root compression. A brain MRI was normal. An EMG/nerve conduction study showed a mild right median mononeuropathy, but no evidence of radiculopathy.

Diagnosis

The following diagnoses were made: (1) periodic arm movements of sleep (PAMS); (2) periodic leg movements of sleep (PLegMS); (3) OSAHS; (4) neck pain; and (5) caffeine abuse.

Follow-up

The patient was CPAP titrated to an optimal pressure of $8\,cmH_2O$; the AHI was reduced to 2 events per hour. Sleep efficiency improved with CPAP.

During follow-up visits, the patient noted a significant improvement in daytime fatigue and sleepiness with the use of CPAP. Sleep quality had also improved, with a reduced number of arousals and wake episodes. Leg and arm movements persisted according to his wife's account. Treatment of the neck/shoulder pain with a muscle relaxant, analgesic and a short course of steroids markedly improved the pain. He worked with occupational therapy and adjusted his work habits to avoid repetitive movements. His use of hydrocodone to relieve the neck and shoulder might have also reduced his periodic arm/leg movements and therefore sleep quality. He was informed of caffeine's negative impact on sleep quality and was advised to reduce consumption.

General remarks

This unique case illustrates a phenomenon that is occasionally encountered during sleep recording: PAMS. Most sleep specialists are more familiar with PLMS occurring in the legs rather than the arms. In part, this may be related to the fact that surface EMG recordings from the arms are not obtained as routinely as those of the tibialis anterior. Additionally, arm movements are not as prominent or do not have as great an amplitude as those seen in the legs. Thus, little is known about PAMS. This patient gave us an opportunity to explore the broader spectrum of sleep-related movement disorder.

Movements of the limbs can occur for a variety of reasons. These disorders can be divided into rhythmical, periodic and random. Rhythmical movements occur in wakefulness or at sleep onset, such as rhythmic movement disorder (RMD), hypnic foot tremor or alternating leg movement activation. Patients are noted to have rocking or head-banging movements occurring prior to sleep onset. Movements are stereotyped; involve large muscles, usually of the head and neck; and are sustained into light sleep. Repetitive behaviors may include head banging (*jactatio capitis nocturna*), body rocking, leg rolling, humming and chanting, and may be more prevalent during periods of emotional stress. The movements are typically more disturbing to the witness than to the patient, but the events can occasionally lead to injury including skull fractures and subdural hematomas. Some patients are unaware of the movements, while others describe the movements as calming. Older patients may experience the motor activity as a compulsion needed to induce sleep. These behaviors are observed in nearly half of infants and 10% of 4-year-olds. The prevalence of the behavior declines with age, being more prevalent in males. Typical episodes on PSG involve rhythmical movements preceding sleep onset and during stage N1 sleep. The key feature of rhythmic movement disorder is the stereotypical/repetitive nature of the behaviors occurring near sleep onset. Episodes may last for minutes to hours and the patient retains consciousness or regains it very rapidly when awakened from sleep. The length of the event and the persistent metronomic feature helps differentiate this disorder from seizure activity.

Hypnic foot tremor is a relatively brief repetitive movement involving one extremity, typically the foot. The movement is characterized by a low-amplitude 0.3–4.0 Hz tremor-like action lasting seconds. The events typically occur near the onset of sleep and may recur throughout the night as the patient transitions from wakefulness to sleep. Most patients are unaware of the movement, but bed partners may notice it. The tremor is not associated with any pathology and does not require treatment.

Alternating leg movement activation (ALMA) is also a benign movement characterized by brief repetitive limb movements similar to those of hypnic foot tremor, but involving alternating limb movement. This feature also differentiates it from the hypnic tremor. The movement occurs at 0.5–3.0 Hz, lasting at least for a set of four movements near sleep onset. These events are benign and do not require treatment. The movements have elements similar to the bicycling motion seen in frontal lobe seizures. However, unlike seizures – which are typically associated with arousal – alternating leg movement activation events occur as a transition to sleep.

Irregular or random motions can be in the form of myoclonus or brief behaviors. Hypnic jerks or sleep starts are quick, brief, sudden movements occurring at sleep onset. These movements may involve any part or all of the body. Virtually everyone experiences these movements, especially when falling asleep in a strange position or after sleep deprivation or emotional stress.

Some patients experience brief sensory phenomena during the event, such as a roaring or buzzing sound, a brief visual scene, a sense of floating or sinking, or pain. Hypnic jerks typically occur at the onset of sleep, rather than at the offset. The lack of a preceding spike discharge helps differentiate hypnic jerks from epileptic myoclonus, and the presence only at sleep onset differentiates hypnic jerks from other myoclonia, which can occur at any time. Hypnic jerks do not require further evaluation or treatment unless the patient snores or displays symptoms of other sleep disorders.

Excessive fragmentary myoclonus consists of single, quick jerks or electromyographic discharges, occurring mostly in NREM sleep. They have a maximal duration of 150 ms and typically have a frequency of more than five events per hour. The movements may not be seen, but can cause twitch-like movements across small joints. Rarely, large joints may be involved. Similar small phasic movements in REM sleep may cause movements across fingers or of facial muscles, and are normal. Excessive fragmentary myoclonus is usually benign and may be differentiated from epileptic myoclonus by the lack of epileptiform discharge on EEG.

Periodic limb movements of sleep are repetitive, stereotyped movements, usually of the lower extremities, typically consisting of extension of the great toe with dorsiflexion of the ankle and flexion of the knee and hip. Some movements may have more of a rotation motion, and movements can involve the arms and axial muscles. The individual movements are brief, lasting 0.5–5 seconds, and occur at 10–90-second intervals. Movements must occur in a set of at least four to be scored as PLMs. Patients are typically unaware of the movements, but bed partners may complain. Movements may seem random, but are shown to be periodic on PSG recording. Only a minority of patients with periodic movements of sleep will have periodic limb movement disorder (PLMD), which includes clinical sequelae such as excessive daytime sleepiness (EDS) or insomnia. In contrast to PLMs, a sensory component is expressed in RLS. Patients note a discomfort with a strong urge to move that is worse during rest, is made better with movement and occurs more frequently in the evening. A majority of, but not all, individuals with RLS have PLMS. These movements are easily distinguished from epileptic phenomena on the basis of their periodic nature and lack of an electroencephalographic correlate. Treatment of PLMs has similarly followed the treatment paradigms of RLS. Dopamine agonists, gabapentin, benzodiazepines and opioids have been used to diminish limb movements. Most of the literature showing these improvements comprises studies involving patients with RLS.

Periodic arm movements of sleep have been reported in a handful of papers. The underyling mechanism of PAMS is unclear and it is unknown whether

PAMS shares the same pathophysiology as periodic leg movements. The generator(s) for these movements are proposed to be in the brainstem or the spinal cord. It has also been proposed that a lesion at these locations acts to release the generator downstream. In our patient, there was no evidence of brainstem or spinal cord lesion; however there was evidence of nerve root irritation on the basis of foraminal stenosis.

The causal relationship between the patient's work-related repetitive arm movements and PAMS is uncertain. However, there was a pattern to his PAMS and PLegMS in respect to their timing during sleep, with the PAMS dominating the early part of his sleep and the PLegMS emerging later. Only one study by Chablis et al. (2000) showed a temporal relationship between PAMS and PLegMS. The arm movements were found to precede leg movements in 41% of cases during wakefulness and in 14% during sleep; however, leg movements were still present during sleep. The cause and mechanism of this temporal relationship is unclear. The presence of PAMS suggests that the structures responsible for generating this periodicity originate at more rostral levels in the neural axis and likely involve the brainstem and other parts of the cortex. Chabli et al. (2000) also showed that PAMs during wakefulness was noted in a large proportion of patients with RLS and that patients with PAMS during wakefulness were more likely to have sleep disturbance.

Arm restlessness is another related phenomenon that needs further exploration. Restless legs syndrome is characterized by leg paresthesias and motor restlessness that leads to discomfort and difficulty with sleep initiation. Symptoms worsen in the evening and at night-time, and are temporarily relieved with movement. Restless legs syndrome is strongly associated with PLMS. Arm restlessness has been reported in nearly half of patients with RLS. Patients who report arm restlessness have severe RLS and worse sleep quality compared with patients without arm restlessness. There is strong evidence implicating the central dopaminergic system and impaired iron processing in RLS and PLMs. It is unknown why either phenomenon tend to predominantly affect the lower limbs.

The treatment of PAMS has not been studied and needs further evaluation. Hydrocodone helped Mr. D. in the relief of his shoulder/neck pain and possibly with the PLMs. Given the high indexes of periodic arm and leg movements during his sleep, it is surprising that the patient did not recount symptoms of RLS. It is possible that hydrocodone had alleviated his restless legs (and possibly restless arms) symptoms. Management of patients with PAMS and restless arms needs to be individualized and, until further research comes along, clinicians can use the PLMs treatment model to help their patients.

Pearls and gold

Periodic limb movements of sleep are repetitive stereotyped movements, usually of the lower extremities, rarely of the arms.

Surface EMG recordings from the arms are not obtained as routinely as from the tibialis anterior, which may hamper knowledge.

Arm movements are not as prominent or do not have as great an amplitude as those seen in the legs.

Management of patients with PAMS and restless arms needs to be individualized and, until further research comes along, clinicians can use the PLMs treatment model to help their patients.

SUGGESTED READING

REVIEWS

Karatas M. Restless legs syndrome and periodic limb movements during sleep: diagnosis and treatment. *Neurologist* 2007; **13**: 294–301.

Walters AS, Lavigne G, Hening W, *et al.* The scoring of movements in sleep. *J Clin Sleep Med* 2007; **3**: 155–67.

GENERAL

AASM (American Academy of Sleep Medicine). *International Classification of Sleep Disorders*, 2nd edn.: *Diagnostic and Coding Manual*. Westchester, Illinois: American Academy of Sleep Medicine, 2005.

AASM (American Academy of Sleep Medicine). *Manual for the Scoring of Sleep and Associated Events: Rules, Terminology and Technical Specification*. Westchester, Illinois: American Academy of Sleep Medicine, 2007.

Chabli A, Michaud M, Montplaisir J. Periodic arm movements in patients with the restless legs syndrome. *Eur Neurol* 2000; **44**: 133–8.

Hoban TF. Rhythmic movement disorder in children. *CNS Spectr* 2003; **8**: 135–8.

Michaud M, Chabli A, Lavigne G, Montplaisir J. Arm restlessness in patients with restless legs syndrome. *Mov Disord* 2000; **15**: 289–93.

Walters AS. Clinical identification of the simple sleep-related movement disorders. *Chest* 2007; **131**: 1260–6.

Yokota T, Shiojiri T, Hirashima F. Sleep-related periodic arm movement. *Sleep* 1995; **18**: 707–8.

Restlessness and jerking upon recumbency when trying to fall asleep

Roberto Vetrugno and Pasquale Montagna

Clinical history

A 56-year-old woman was admitted to hospital after a 2-year history of uncomfortable sensations with pain and paresthesia accompanied by an urge to move the legs at rest upon recumbency, especially in the evening and at night. In the last year, involuntary jerks of the trunk and limbs had appeared, arising repetitively when she was awake and lying supine and co-existing with motor restlessness, together causing difficulties in initiating and maintaining sleep and resulting in complaints of excessive daytime sleepiness (EDS) and tiredness. Her past medical history included tension headaches. There was no family history of movement disorders.

Examination

A neurological examination showed generalized increased deep tendon reflexes, but plantar responses were flexor. Her average resting systemic blood pressure was 120/70 mmHg and her heart rate was 68 bpm. Sudden acoustic, visual and tactile (glabella tapping) stimuli did not evoke any abnormal motor phenomena. A neuropsychological assessment, including the mini mental state examination, was normal. Routine blood analyses including a complete blood count, creatinine, electrolytes, liver enzymes, bilirubin, uric acid, lactate dehydrogenase, glucose, iron, ferritin and thyroid function were normal. Brain and spinal cord MRIs were normal.

Special studies

Electrophysiological investigation was performed by means of electromyography and electroneurography (EMG-ENG) and visual, brainstem auditory, motor and somatosensory evoked potentials, the latter combined with recording of long latency EMG responses (C reflex) and blink reflexes. Thereafter, the patient

Case Studies in Sleep Neurology: Common and Uncommon Presentations, ed. A. Culebras. Published by Cambridge University Press. © Cambridge University Press 2010.

underwent all-night video-polysomnography (PSG) recordings by means of a 21-channel Grass polygraph connected to a computerized system (Neuroscan; Herndon) for off-line analysis of acquired data (16-bit resolution, sampling rate 1024 Hz; EEG bandpass 0.1–60 Hz; EMG bandpass 50–300 Hz). EMG activity was recorded from various facial, neck, trunk and upper and lower limb muscles.

Question

How would you categorize this movement disorder?

Results of studies

The neurophysiological and video-PSG test results as well as the EMG-ENG, visual, brainstem auditory, motor and somatosensory evoked potentials, and blink reflex were all normal. Long latency EMG responses (C reflex) were absent.

Video-PSG demonstrated motor restlessness during relaxed wakefulness preceding sleep onset and during wakefulness after sleep onset: the patient repetitively stretched and flexed the legs and often shifted body posture. At the same time, she reported an uncomfortable and "inside" sensation causing an urge to move the legs with partial/total, but only momentary, relief brought about by moving the legs. In addition, during relaxed wakefulness, flexion jerks of the trunk co-existed with the motor restlessness and sensory discomfort in the limbs. During a single recording, 52 such jerks were recorded, occurring in isolation or in a repetitive manner (Figure 36.1).

The EMG of these axial jerks was characterized by discharges starting in the right intercostalis muscle with subsequent involvement of other trunkal, lower limb and neck muscles. The EMG discharges lasted 200–500 ms, but sometimes longer with polymyoclonic shape, and manifested both reciprocal and co-contracting

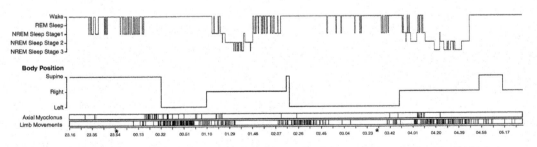

Figure 36.1 Sleep histogram showing the occurrence of axial myoclonus and periodic limb movements of sleep (PLMS) in relation to the sleep/wake cycle and body position. Asterisks indicates transient suppression of axial myoclonus by mental exercise.

(a)

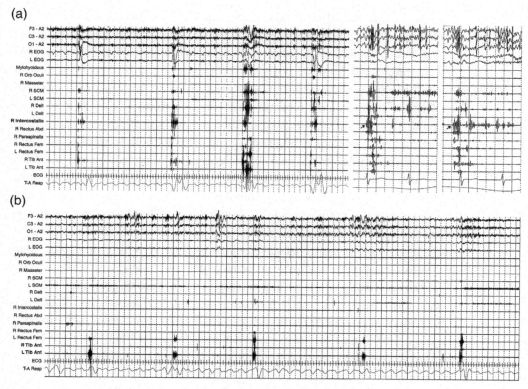

(b)

Figure 36.2 (a) Polygraphic recordings showing multiple episodes of axial myoclonus during relaxed wakefulness (left panel; paper speed 10 mm/s) with a rostrocaudal propagation of muscular activity starting in the intercostalis muscle (right panel; dotted line; paper speed 30 mm/s) and spreading to rostral and caudal muscles in a manner typical of propriospinal myoclonus. (b) Polygraphic recordings during NREM sleep showing PLMS involving the tibialis anterior muscles only, with a characteristic periodicity of 20–40 seconds (paper speed 10 mm/s). EOG, electro-oculogram; Orb Oculi, orbicularis oculi; SCM, sternocleidomastoideus; Delt, deltoideus; Rectus Abd, rectus abdominis; Rectus Fem, rectus femoris; Tib Ant, tibialis anterior; ECG, electrocardiogram; T-A Resp, thoraco-abdominal respirogram; R, right; L, left.

agonist–antagonist activity. Jitter occurred from jerk to jerk with regard to the relative timing of the various EMG discharges within each episode of myoclonus (Figure 36.2). The delay between the first activated (i.e. intercostalis) and the most caudal (i.e. tibialis anterior) and rostral (i.e. sternocleidomastoideus) muscles was 25–120 ms, giving a spinal conduction velocity of 3–12 m/s (crudely obtained by first measuring the distance between the vertebral level corresponding to the myotome of the starting muscle and the rostral [C1] and caudal [L2] limits of the spinal cord, and then dividing this distance by the time delays of the rostral-most and caudal-most activated muscles). No EEG correlates in the routine recording or upon jerk-related EEG-EMG back-averaging were disclosed. This axial myoclonic activity appeared during relaxed wakefulness when EEG alpha rhythm spread from the posterior to the anterior cortical areas or when it dropped out during stage N1 sleep. Jerks could recur at quasi-periodic intervals (every 10–50 seconds) and repeated themselves associated with delayed sleep onset and sleep fragmentation. Remarkably, mental activation with the patient comfortably lying down or sitting (asking the patient to think, speak, count and perform simple motor tasks such as making a fist) desynchronized the EEG activity and at the same time made the axial jerks disappear. Axial myoclonus thereafter reappeared as soon as the patient was left undisturbed and relaxed, and EEG alpha activity again spread or dropped out. The axial jerks, however, disappeared with sleep onset (i.e. with the appearance of the sleep spindles and K-complexes) and were not observed during sleep, at which time they were replaced by typical periodic limb movements of sleep (PLMS) with EMG activity now restricted mainly to the tibialis anterior muscle (Figures 36.1 and 36.2).

There was a significant sleep fragmentation with decreased sleep efficiency (31%; normal value ≥85%) and reduced total sleep time (TST: 115 minutes; sleep stages: 44% stage N1, 38% stage N2, 18% stages N3–N4, 0% REM sleep; wakefulness after sleep onset: 200 minutes). The mean arousal index was 37 per hour, mean periodic limb movement index while awake (PLMA) was 40 per hour and mean PLMS index was 51 per hour. Clonazepam 2 mg at night was started and was reported as effective in reducing the jerks and in mitigating motor restlessness before sleep onset, thus allowing the patient to fall asleep.

Follow-up

The patient reported a 2-year history of urge to move the legs accompanied by an uncomfortable and unpleasant sensation in the legs, appearing during rest, relieved with movement and worsening during the evening/night-time. These features fit the ICSD-2 (AASM, 2005) criteria for restless legs syndrome (RLS). Additionally, involuntary trunk jerks preceding falling asleep and during intrasleep wakefulness appeared during the disease progression, bothersome to the patient and impeding falling asleep. Neurophysiology confirmed that these axial jerks occurred solely at the transition from wakefulness to sleep, during intrasleep arousal and upon awakening, i.e. when the patient was relaxed but awake. The diffusion of the jerks to involve multiple spinal segments, their origin in the intercostalis muscles, the long duration of the EMG bursts (200–500 ms or longer), the jitter in intermuscle latencies and the low spinal conduction velocity are all characteristics of myoclonus of propriospinal origin, i.e. propriospinal myoclonus (PSM).

Diagnosis

The diagnosis was idiopathic RLS and PSM.

General remarks

Absence of a cortical pre-movement potential and lack of involvement of cranial muscles distinguish PSM from cortical and reticular reflex myoclonus. Remarkably, PSM in our patient was observed to flare up at the transition from wakefulness to sleep and did not seem to relate only to the recumbency posture, but rather to vigilance level. Indeed, the jerks could be promptly abolished by mental activation, even with the patient lying down, and immediately restarted when the patient was left alone undisturbed. Jerks arose during relaxed wakefulness when EEG alpha activity spread from posterior occipital to anterior frontal areas, and disappeared again with sleep onset (spindles and/or K-complexes) and throughout sleep proper when PSM was replaced by PLMS with a different motor pattern of activation, now limited to the muscles of the lower limbs, especially the tibialis anterior.

Propriospinal myoclonus has been described as an isolated finding occurring at the transition from wakefulness to sleep, and causing insomnia. In the original reports, PSM occurred in the absence of other neurological disturbances or, more rarely, associated with spinal cord lesions. The case that we report here emphasizes how PSM may also occur in the context of idiopathic RLS, and how it should be kept distinct from the PLMS typically associated with RLS because of its specific time window of appearance and pattern of muscular propagation. Propriospinal myoclonus at the wake/sleep transition is not, however, a recognized clinical feature contemplated in the criteria necessary for the diagnosis of RLS.

Other clinical entities entering the differential diagnosis of these axial jerks are the focal abnormal involuntary movements of the abdominal wall reported under the terms "diaphragmatic flutter," "moving umbilicus syndrome" and "belly dancer's dyskinesia," which have different clinical features and EMG patterns from those observed in our patient, consisting of irregular or writhing contractions of the affected muscles at rates as high as 30–90 per minute and involving the diaphragmatic or abdominal muscles as a focal rather than propagated form.

Painful legs and moving toes identifies a condition characterized by severe pain of the feet with a burning sensation and repetitive semicontinuous movements of the toes, with irregular EMG bursts in the small muscles of the foot and leg and not necessarily worsening at night or relieved by activity, which is thus completely different for location and pattern from PSM.

Excessive fragmentary hypnic myoclonus refers to the muscular twitches involving the fingers, toes and corners of the mouth, persisting in all stages of sleep and whose EMG findings resemble fasciculation potentials and/or the phasic REM twitches that are a normal finding in REM sleep, except that they persist in all sleep stages and are not clustered in REM sleep.

Sleep starts are non-periodic myoclonic movements, usually involving asynchronically different and isolated body segments as a normal accompaniment of sleep and associated with a K-complex or EEG arousal. Sleep starts have been reported to cause insomnia when intensified; however, they do not primarily involve the abdominal muscles.

In conclusion, several kinds of motor activity were observed in this patient (RLS dyskinesia, PSM and PLMS) with different motor patterns and recurrence during different states of vigilances. At the wake/sleep transition, PSM displays a peculiar relationship with the states of vigilance, recurring only upon relaxation and drowsiness, i.e. the so-called pre-dormitum. The peculiar time relationship between PSM and PLMS (PSM disappears with sleep onset, when PLMS in turn arises) has led to the hypothesis that one movement becomes transformed into the other when supraspinal dysfacilitatory influences typical of the wake/sleep transition responsible for the PSM change to light sleep and consequently to the PLMS.

The clinician and sleep specialist should be alert to the possibility that RLS and PSM may occur together in a still unspecified percentage of cases. It is also relevant that, in our patient, axial jerks were reported as uncomfortable and as sleep disturbing as the paresthesia and motor restlessness of RLS, while PLMS went unheeded by the patient. These axial jerks justified the administration of clonazepam, which was reported as useful, even though dopaminergic medications represent the first choice in RLS therapy. Whether indeed PSM responds to dopaminergic therapy is still unknown.

Finally we caution that the presence of PSM in the course of RLS may easily be missed if PSG recordings are run with an EMG montage restricted to the leg muscles only and not involving also the axial trunkal/abdominal muscles.

Pearls and gold

Restless legs syndrome and PSM may occur together.

Propriospinal myoclonus displays a peculiar relationship with the states of vigilance, recurring only upon relaxation and drowsiness, i.e. the so-called pre-dormitum.

Propriospinal myoclonus in the course of RLS may easily be missed if PSG recordings are run without involving axial trunkal and abdominal muscles.

Clonazepam has been reported as useful in the control of PSM.

SUGGESTED READING

HISTORICAL

Montagna P, Provini F, Plazzi G, Liguori R, Lugaresi E. Propriospinal myoclonus upon relaxation and drowsiness: a cause of severe insomnia. *Mov Disord* 1997; **12**: 66–72.

REVIEW

Montagna P, Provini F, Vetrugno R. Propriospinal myoclonus at sleep onset. *Neurophysiol Clin* 2006; **36**: 351–5.

GENERAL

AASM (American Academy of Sleep Medicine). *International Classification of Sleep Disorders*, 2nd edn.: *Diagnostic and Coding Manual*. Westchester, Illinois: American Academy of Sleep Medicine, 2005.

Montagna P. Sleep-related non epileptic motor disorders. *J Neurol* 2004; **251**: 781–94.

Vetrugno R, Provini F, Meletti S, *et al.* Propriospinal myoclonus at the sleep-wake transition: a new type of parasomnia. *Sleep* 2001; **24**: 835–43.

Vetrugno R, Provini F, Plazzi G, Cortelli P, Montagna P. Propriospinal myoclonus: a motor phenomenon found in restless legs syndrome different from periodic limb movements during sleep. *Mov Disord* 2005; **10**: 1323–9.

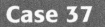

Jumping and yelling while asleep

Rosalia C. Silvestri

Clinical history

Mr. Y. had come to the sleep clinic accompanied by his wife who reported that her husband was very restless and kept jerking all night long from the moment he fell asleep. He often screamed, wept or mumbled incomprehensible words and on a few occasions, most recently, would yell at her and punch her in his sleep. No dreams were reported upon spontaneous or provoked awakenings. This had been going on since the death of his mother, 2 years ago. Mr. Y. complained of having a hard time going to sleep because of unrelenting jerks involving his limbs and shoulders the moment he fell asleep and having the sensation of sinking into a void. The patient also reported frequent palpitations, precordialgia with a negative cardiology workout, anxiety and hypomnesia, but no excessive daytime sleepiness (EDS).

Examination

The neurologist in sleep disorders evaluating Mr. Y. elicited a normal physical and neurological examination.

Special studies

The neurologist ordered nocturnal video-polysomnography (PSG) to include several proximal as well as distal limb muscles and an eight-lead EEG recording, as well as standard sleep parameters.

Question

Does this patient have nocturnal seizures or REM-sleep behavior disorder (RBD)?

Case Studies in Sleep Neurology: Common and Uncommon Presentations, ed. A. Culebras. Published by Cambridge University Press. © Cambridge University Press 2010.

Follow-up

The specialist asked Mr. Y. if he had ever had seizures as a child, an abnormal EEG recording or sustained a head trauma, eliciting negative answers to all questions. He also asked whether he suffered as a child from sleepwalking, night terrors, enuresis, bruxism or any other unusual phenomena during his sleep. Once again, he obtained a negative reply. Lastly, he asked whether he had felt awkward or slowed down lately in his movements and daily activities or whether he had any relatives diagnosed with Parkinson's disease. No such cases were reported.

Results of studies

Mr. Y.'s PSG results showed very superficial and fragmented sleep, with a sleep efficiency of 38%. Several bouts of snoring activity were recorded dispersed in all stages of sleep, but no apneas were detected. Hypnic myoclonus was also recorded in brief, fragmentary sequences involving the trunk and four limbs in all stages of sleep, more so at the beginning of the night accompanied by somniloquy or yelling (Figure 37.1). Throughout the night, more complex random gesturing appeared with elaborate talking. REM sleep showed physiological tone

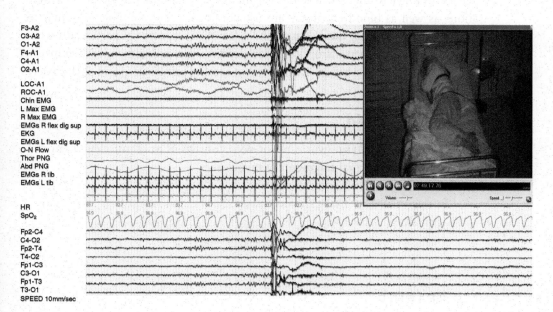

Figure 37.1 Sleep starts in sleep transition. LOC/ROC, left/right outer canthus; flex dig sup, flexor digitorum superior; O-N Flow, oral–nasal flow; Thor, thorax; Abd, abdomen; PNG, pneumograph; tib, tibialis; HR, heart rate.

suppression, albeit with persistence of fragmentary myoclonus. Periodic leg movements with pathological significance were not recorded.

Diagnosis

On the basis of PSG, the specialist made a diagnosis of excessive fragmentary myoclonus and sleep starts. The patient received a recommendation to start clonazepam 1 mg before sleep and he was also prescribed sertraline 50 mg daily for chronic anxiety disorder. A follow-up visit was scheduled in 2 months.

General remarks

Excessive fragmentary myoclonus is a variant of "normal" fragmentary myoclonus, occurring predominantly in males, with a relatively benign course suggesting that it is not associated with a neurodegenerative disease, but may rather be due to disruptions of normal motor control mechanisms in sleep. It consists of asymmetrical, asynchronous, brief jerks involving various muscles of the face, trunk, arms and legs in all sleep stages, persisting during REM sleep. In contrast, bilaterally synchronous and larger myoclonic movements at sleep onset characterize "sleep starts," which are generally known to affect both genders at any age. Physical and neurological examinations as well as blood chemistry are usually normal. Polysomnography may be requested only to clarify the diagnosis and rule out seizure activity, particularly when there is consistent sleep disruption. Clonazepam is the recommended therapeutic strategy aiming to relieve excessive movement activity, restore sleep and quell anxiety.

Pearls and gold

Excessive fragmentary myoclonus of sleep consists of brief muscle jerks and is a variant of normal fragmentary myoclonus.

It occurs predominantly in males.

Excessive fragmentary myoclonus is a benign condition but may disrupt sleep.

SUGGESTED READING

HISTORICAL

Oswald I. Sudden bodily jerks on falling asleep. *Brain* 1959; **82**: 92–103.

REVIEW

Walters AS, Lavigne G, Hening W, *et al.* The scoring of movements in sleep. *J Clin Sleep Med* 2007; **3**: 155–67.

GENERAL

AASM (American Academy of Sleep Medicine). *International Classification of Sleep Disorders*, 2nd edn.: *Diagnostic and Coding Manual.* Westchester, Illinois: American Academy of Sleep Medicine, 2005.

Broughton R. Pathological fragmentary myoclonus, intensified sleep starts and hypnagogic foot tremor: three unusual sleep related disorders. In: Koella WP, Obal F, Schulz H, Wisser P, eds. *Sleep 86, Proceedings of the Eighth European Congress on Sleep Research*, Szeged Hungary, September 1986. New York: Fisher Verlag; 1988: 240–3.

Lins O, Castonguay M, Dunham W, Nevsimalova S, Broughton R. Excessive fragmentary myoclonus: time of night and sleep stage distributions. *Can J Neurol Sci* 1993; **20**: 142–6.

Sander HW, Geisse H, Quinto C, Sachdeo R, Chokroverty S. Sensory sleep starts. *J Neurol Neurosurg Psychiatry* 1998; **64**: 690.

Case 38

A case of attention deficit

David E. McCarty

Clinical history

Thomas was 6 years old and uncontrollable. His teachers complained that he was easily distractable, with impulsive and hyperactive behavior. Concerns over poor academic progress led to psychiatric evaluation and a diagnosis of attention deficit hyperactivity disorder (ADHD) was made. He did not tolerate stimulant medication, primarily due to worsening problems with sleep-onset and sleep-maintenance insomnia, which had been present essentially since birth. His mother reported that he had always been difficult to put to bed and that he frequently got into trouble for repeatedly getting out of bed and waking her up. He had previously been a heavy snorer, but had undergone an adenotonsillectomy at the age of 4 years, which improved (but did not eliminate) his snoring.

In an effort to treat the ADHD with associated sleep disturbance, his physician recommended clonidine, which initially helped with his sleep-onset insomnia, but which later lost effect. Quetiapine was added, which, according to his mother, dramatically improved his ability to fall asleep, and allowed approximately 4 or 5 hours of relative sleep continuity, after which he would waken frequently. Shortly after Thomas started the quetiapine, however, his teachers called his mother with complaints about him falling asleep in class. A sleep medicine consultation was requested for further evaluation.

On questioning, Thomas revealed that he always had a sense of discomfort in his legs, or, as he described it, "like ants crawling under my skin" when he was at rest. He reported that these symptoms seemed to improve as long as he was moving his legs and were always more intense at night. His mother corroborated that, even during sleep, Thomas "always seemed to be moving." On further questioning, Thomas's mother reported that she had suffered from similar symptoms since early adulthood.

Case Studies in Sleep Neurology: Common and Uncommon Presentations, ed. A. Culebras. Published by Cambridge University Press. © Cambridge University Press 2010.

Examination

Thomas was found to be a well-developed, thin, but healthy appearing boy, sniffling during the interview and mouth breathing. His height was 110 cm (50th percentile) and weight 20 kg (25th percentile). A nasal examination revealed mucosal edema and poor nasal airflow without turbinate hypertrophy or polyps. Cardiopulmonary and neurological examinations were unremarkable. Behaviorally, he was very hyperactive, with evidence of impulsivity, including frequent interruptions of conversations and inappropriately rough climbing activity throughout the examination room, requiring repeated parental interventions.

Preliminary remarks

The diagnosis of ADHD is often based upon the DSM-IV criteria (American Psychiatric Association, 2000), with clinical descriptions of behaviors reflecting developmentally inappropriate functional impairment of attention, impulsivity and hyperactivity, in the absence of an underlying mood or mental disorder to better explain the symptoms. Although sleep deprivation is commonly understood to result in cognitive and behavioral symptoms that overlap with ADHD, treatable sleep disorders often go unrecognized in children with these symptoms, leading to erroneous diagnosis. In fact, sleep disturbances are so commonly recognized to be part of the clinical spectrum of ADHD that nocturnal sleep disruption used to be included in the diagnostic criteria. The frequent association of sleep disruption with ADHD may result in physician complacency when troubled sleep is part of the presentation of ADHD-like behaviors, leading to the failure to further investigate subjective sleep disturbances in these children.

Questions

1. What sleep-related diagnoses are most appropriate?
2. What testing, if any, should be requested?
3. What medication changes, if any, should be recommended?
4. Does this patient truly have ADHD?

Special studies

Nocturnal polysomnography (PSG) and a serum ferritin test were ordered.

Results of studies

His serum ferritin was 29 ng/ml. Typically, a value of ≤50 ng/mL is considered a marker for systemic iron deficiency and suggests potential benefit for replacement.

Polysomnography (done with the patient still taking clonidine and quetiapine) showed early sleep latency (the patient was asleep at lights out) with reduced REM sleep (12% of total sleep time [TST]) and higher-than-expected values for slow-wave sleep (37% of TST). Sleep fragmentation was seen with an arousal index of 13 per hour of sleep. Leg movements were noted to occur throughout the study, both during periods of recorded sleep and wakefulness. The periodic limb movement (PLM) index was 22 per hour of sleep. Respiratory monitoring revealed the presence of mild snoring and upper-airway resistance features, but no significant apneas or hypopneas. The total sleep time apnea–hypopnea index (AHI) was 0.1 per hour of sleep. The minimum O_2 saturation was 96%.

Follow-up

Iron supplementation was recommended and quetiapine was discontinued. Medical management of allergic rhinitis was begun with montelukast and cetirizine, with improvement in nocturnal snoring observed by the patient's mother. Specific treatment for restless legs syndrome (RLS) was instituted. An initial trial on clonazepam produced suboptimal symptomatic improvement at low dose (0.125 mg at bedtime) and next-day drowsiness when the dose was increased. Clonazepam was discontinued, and pramipexole 0.125 mg, taken an hour before bedtime, was started. Subsequently, a dramatic improvement in the patient's subjective leg discomfort, as well as an improvement in sleep-onset and sleep-maintenance insomnia, was noted. An attempt to discontinue clonidine resulted in a return of sleep-onset insomnia, and this medication was subsequently restarted.

The patient was seen regularly in follow-up for the next several months during the period of medication adjustment, and frequent telephone contacts were made. At a follow-up appointment 6 months after his initial diagnostic PSG, the patient's mother reported that she rated her satisfaction with her son's sleeping patterns as "without question, a 10 on a 10-point scale." The patient had no difficulty initiating or maintaining sleep. In addition, his school performance improved dramatically, qualifying him for the gifted and talented program, and earning him a citizenship award for exemplary classroom behavior.

At his follow-up interview, the patient was talkative and enthusiastic, but did not interrupt conversations, and sat patiently on the examination table while the physician and his mother discussed his progress.

Diagnosis

The following diagnoses were made: (1) childhood-onset RLS and periodic limb movement disorder (PLMD); (2) iron deficiency; (3) hypersomnia due to drug/ substance (quetiapine); and (4) allergic/chronic rhinitis with snoring and upper- airway resistance features.

General remarks

Thomas had classic clinical symptoms of RLS: irritable discomfort in the legs brought on by rest, provoking an urge to move the legs, which resulted in temporary relief of the symptoms. His symptoms also exhibited diurnal variation, with worse symptoms at night. Restless legs syndrome is a movement disorder resulting from decreased regional central nervous system dopamine, a neuro- transmitter that requires an iron-dependent enzyme (tyrosine hydroxylase) for the first, rate-limiting step in its synthesis. As a result, iron deficiency can result in clinical RLS in susceptible individuals. Restless legs syndrome is tightly linked to iron deficiency, particularly in children, with low serum ferritin (≤ 50 ng/ml) found in as many as 83% of children with RLS. A genetic susceptibility for RLS is suspected and, in children, RLS in a first-degree relative is also supportive of the diagnosis. Childhood-onset RLS can be misdiagnosed as "growing pains" or remain unsuspected due to a child's poor ability to verbalize the symptoms. The symptoms can be potentiated by many classes of medication, including many antidepressants (selective serotonin reuptake inhibitors and tricyclic antidepres- sants) and antipsychotics. In this case, it is conceivable that Thomas's symptoms and sleep fragmentation (from periodic limb movements of sleep) could ironic- ally have been accentuated by the quetiapine, ostensibly prescribed to improve the quality of his sleep.

Thomas's snoring also deserves further consideration. Snoring in children is independently associated with future risk of hyperactive behavior. It is conceiv- able that respiratory disturbances could be stimulating Thomas's "constant movement" during sleep, noted by his mother. This child had already under- gone adenotonsillectomy, a procedure that often (but not always) resolves sleep- disordered breathing in children. If Thomas were found to have significant sleep apnea, further treatment measures might be necessary, such as medical or surgical management of obstructive nasal conditions, oral–maxillofacial surgical procedures, orthodontic appliances or continuous positive airway pressure (CPAP).

Given the resolution of Thomas's attention-deficit, hyperactivity, and impulsivity symptoms following specific treatment for his sleep disorders, the diagnosis of ADHD was abandoned. It was later remarked that Thomas's case is quite instructive, and may serve to prevent physicians from having "attention deficit" to sleep-specific complaints in children, allowing more accurate diagnoses and more effective treatments.

Pearls and gold

The frequent association of sleep disruption with ADHD may result in physician complacency when troubled sleep is part of the presentation of ADHD-like behaviors, leading to the failure to further investigate subjective sleep disturbances in these children.

Restless legs syndrome may lurk behind symptoms of hyperactivity, impulsivity and altered sleep in children with "growing pains" and other manifestations of leg discomfort.

Restless legs syndrome is tightly linked to iron deficiency in many children. Low serum ferritin ($\leq$50 ng/ml) is found in as many as 83% children with RLS. Management with pramipexole is also gratifying in children with RLS.

SUGGESTED READING

HISTORICAL

Ekbom KA. Asthenia crurum paraesthetica ("Irritable Legs"). A new syndrome consisting of weakness, sensation of cold and nocturnal paraesthesia in the legs, responding to a certain extent to treatment in general. *Acta Med Scand* 1944; **118**: 197–209.

Ekbom KA. Restless legs. *JAMA* 1946; **131**: 481–6.

Ekbom KA. Growing pains and restless legs. *Acta Paediatr Scand* 1975; **64**: 264–6.

REVIEW

Allen RP, Picchietti D, Hening WA, *et al*. Restless legs syndrome: diagnostic criteria, special considerations, and epidemiology. A report from the restless legs syndrome diagnosis and epidemiology workshop at the National Institutes of Health. *Sleep Med* 2003; **4**: 101–19.

GENERAL

American Psychiatric Association. *Diagnostic and Statistical Manual of Mental Disorders, Text Revision (DSM IV-TR)*. Washington, DC: American Psychiatric Association, 2000.

Chervin RD, Ruzicka DL, Archbold KH, *et al*. Snoring predicts hyperactivity four years later. *Sleep* 2005; **28**: 885–90.

Kotagal S, Silber MH. (2004). Childhood-onset restless legs syndrome. *Ann Neurol* **56**: 803–7.

Ondo WG. Iron deficiency-associated restless legs syndrome. In: Ondo WG, ed. *Restless Legs Syndrome: Diagnosis and Treatment*. New York, NY: Informa Healthcare USA, 2008; 211–18.

Owens JA. The ADHD and sleep conundrum: a review. *J Devel Behav Ped* 2005; **26**: 312–22.

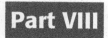
Part VIII

Neuromuscular disorders and sleep

Snoring and leg cramps

Antonio Culebras

Clinical history

Mr. P. had been tested in another laboratory and was told that he had sleep apnea. He received a continuous positive airway pressure (CPAP) device, but abandoned its use some time later. At the age of 57 years, he came to the sleep center complaining of snoring louder than before the first test had been done and of leg cramps. He usually went to bed at 10 pm, falling asleep 30 minutes later. He would remain asleep all night except for two short awakenings to urinate. The wife reported that his snoring was very loud, so loud that it could be heard outside the bedroom. In addition, she had observed lapses in respiratory activity, particularly when Mr. P. slept on his back. Mr. P. also complained of occasional cramps in both legs that would wake him up. At least on three occasions, he had dreamt that an attacker was chasing him and ended the episode waking up with his hands around the neck of his startled wife. His wake-up time had generally been around 8 am, commonly feeling tired and at times complaining of a headache that would dissipate shortly thereafter. Typically, he was sleepy during the day and took 3-hour naps without dream content. His Epworth Sleepiness Scale score was 11, which suggested only mild sleepiness (see Appendix).

His past history was relevant for a diagnosis of primary lateral sclerosis that had been made 12 years before. He also had systemic hypertension, a history of pulmonary embolus and frequent headaches. He had undergone lumbar laminectomy and several orthopedic operations in his lower extremities. He was taking gabapentin, fluoxetine, lisinopril, modafinil, baclofen and warfarin. His family history was negative for neurological and sleep disorders.

Examination

The examination showed a well-developed man with normal higher mental function. Cranial nerve testing was normal. Motor power in the upper extremities

Case Studies in Sleep Neurology: Common and Uncommon Presentations, ed. A. Culebras. Published by Cambridge University Press. © Cambridge University Press 2010.

was normal, but in the lower extremities there was mild distal weakness with mildly increased muscle tone. Deep tendon reflexes were symmetrical and increased in both lower extremities. Responses to plantar stimulation were mute. His sensory perception was normal. His gait was typically paraparetic with inability to walk on his heels or toes.

Examination of the oropharynx revealed a small Mallampati class 3 space. His pulse was regular at 70 bpm and his blood pressure was 145/98 mmHg. His height was 171.5 cm and weight 88 kg, with a BMI of 29.9 kg/m^2.

Special studies

A polysomnography (PSG) study was performed with the sleep apnea protocol and video recording. This was followed 10 days later by a positive airway pressure (PAP) protocol study.

Question

What is your diagnosis?

Results of studies

The sleep study was predictably abnormal because of the presence of sleep apnea. Apneas were of the obstructive, non-obstructive and mixed varieties. Apnea events were more abundant with more arousals and desaturations while the patient slept supine (Figure 39.1). The apnea–hypopnea index (AHI) overall was 33.2 events per hour and 59.4 while sleeping supine. The hemoglobin O$_2$ saturation nadir while sleeping supine was 80%. Periodic breathing and Cheyne–Stokes respirations were also identified. However periodic limb movements, REM sleep without atonia and abnormal nocturnal behaviors were not observed. Sleep stages were otherwise normal with an average sleep latency of 22 minutes and a REM-sleep latency of 157 minutes. A subsequent sleep study with the PAP protocol showed a favorable response to the application of CPAP at 9 cmH$_2$O pressure with an excellent tolerance (Figure 39.2).

Diagnosis

The diagnosis was positional sleep apnea of moderate to severe intensity in a patient with primary lateral sclerosis, together with REM-sleep behavior disorder (RBD) by history.

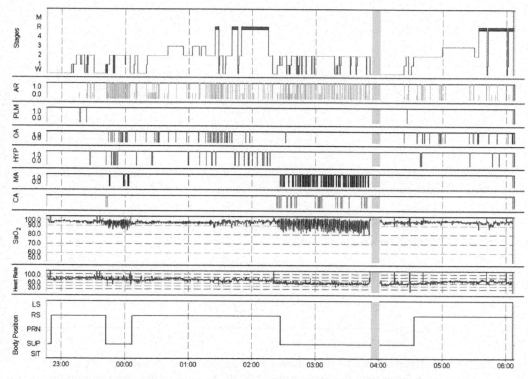

Figure 39.1 Hypnogram showing sleep hypopnea and apnea events of the obstructive, non-obstructive, central and mixed variety with aggravation in the supine position in NREM sleep. Stages: W, wakefulness; R, REM; M, movement; AR, arousals. PLM, periodic leg movements; OA, obstructive apneas; HYP, hypopneas; MA, mixed apneas; CA, central apneas; SaO_2, hemoglobin saturation of O_2. Body position: LS, left side; RS, right side; PRN, prone; SUP, supine.

General remarks

Mr. P. was afflicted with primary lateral sclerosis, a slowly progressive non-inherited gait disorder that may show no abnormalities on examination other than signs implicating the corticospinal tracts. Primary lateral sclerosis is a diagnosis of exclusion, proven only at autopsy. Modern technology can exclude other disorders that can cause the syndrome including compressive lesions at the foramen magnum or cervical spinal cord, multiple sclerosis, amyotrophic lateral sclerosis, Chiari malformation, syringomyelia, biochemical abnormality and persistent infection with human immunodeficiency virus or human T-lymphotrophic virus type I.

Many patients with neurodegenerative disorder and certainly most patients with neuromuscular disorder, if they live long enough, will develop a sleep-related

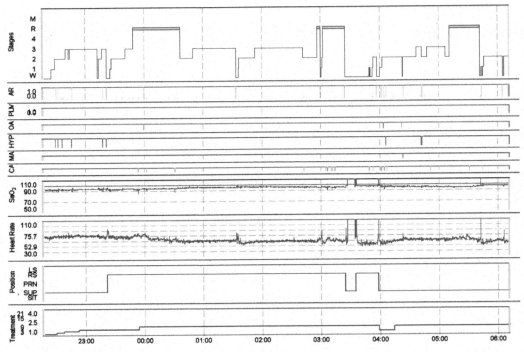

Figure 39.2 Virtual disappearance of sleep apnea and hypopnea events with correction of O_2 saturation levels with the application of CPAP. A modest REM-sleep rebound is observed. Stages: W, wakefulness; R, REM; M, movement; AR, arousals; PLM, periodic leg movements; OA, obstructive apneas; HYP, hypopneas; MA, mixed apneas; CA, central apneas; SaO_2, hemoglobin saturation of O_2. Body position: LS, left side; RS, right side; PRN, prone; SUP, supine.

breathing disorder, either sleep apnea or hypoventilation–hyposaturation disorder. These are classified in ICSD-2 (AASM, 2005) as sleep-related hypoventilation/hypoxemia, due to neuromuscular and chest-wall disorders under the heading "Sleep-related hypoventilation/hypoxemia due to medical conditions" in the larger category of "Sleep-related breathing disorders." Primary lateral sclerosis likely involves muscles of the oropharynx. It is conceivable that, while sleeping supine, the oropharyngeal space is reduced even further because of the weight of the tongue, which cannot be maintained in place due to weakness of the oropharyngeal muscles. This is a plausible mechanism of sleep apnea aggravation in patients with neuromuscular disorders. Fortunately, the response to CPAP or bilevel PAP is generally very favorable, improving the quality of life, although not modifying the natural progression of the underlying neurological disorder.

In addition, our patient had a clinical history suggestive of RBD. This condition facilitates the enactment of dreams when muscle tone fails to decrease in REM sleep. It is a common occurrence in central neurodegenerative disorders. Although not described in primary lateral sclerosis, RBD has been reported in disorders of central neurodegeneration, particularly when affecting the brainstem.

On follow-up 3 months later, Mr. P. was tolerating the CPAP device and doing well in general. His snoring had disappeared and daytime sleepiness was less severe. Lower extremity weakness remained unchanged and further episodes of enactment of dreams had not occurred, suggesting that perhaps uncontrolled sleep apnea had precipitated the episodes of RBD.

Pearls and gold

Most patients with neuromuscular disorder, if they live long enough, will develop a sleep-related breathing disorder, either sleep apnea or hypoventilation–hyposaturation disorder.

Primary lateral sclerosis likely involves muscles of the oropharynx causing or aggravating sleep apnea.

The response to CPAP or bilevel PAP is generally very favorable, improving the quality of life, although not modifying the natural progression of the underlying neurological disorder.

SUGGESTED READING

HISTORICAL

Schenck CH, Bundlie SR, Ettinger MG, Mahowald MW. Chronic behavioral disorders of human REM sleep: a new category of parasomnia. *Sleep* 1986; **9**: 293–308.

REVIEW

Mahowald MW, Schenck CH. REM sleep behavior disorder. In Culebras A, ed. *Sleep Disorders and Neurological Diseases*, 2nd edn. New York: Informa Healthcare USA, 2007; 263–75.

GENERAL

AASM (American Academy of Sleep Medicine). *International Classification of Sleep Disorders*, 2nd edn.: *Diagnostic and Coding Manual*. Westchester, Illinois: American Academy of Sleep Medicine, 2005.

Culebras A. Sleep-disordered breathing in neuromuscular disease. *Sleep Med Clin* 2008; **3**: 377–86.

Gordon PH, Cheng B, Katz IB, *et al.* The natural history of primary lateral sclerosis. *Neurology* 2006; **66**: 647–53.

Younger DS, Chou S, Hays AP, *et al.* Primary lateral sclerosis. A clinical diagnosis reemerges. *Arch Neurol* 1988; **45**: 1304–7.

"So tired I take naps in the morning"

Antonio Culebras

Clinical history

Mr. F. was a 37-year-old man referred to the sleep center for evaluation of excessive daytime fatigue and sleepiness that had been present for several years. His referring physician had suspected sleep apnea. He generally went to bed between 11 pm and 2 am and fell asleep 20 minutes later. At times, there was discomfort in his legs that delayed the onset of sleep. According to the wife, he snored loudly and had exhibited lapses in respiratory activity of which the patient was unaware. He was restless while asleep, but had not fallen out of bed. Numbness in the extremities and discomfort in the legs would wake him up at night. His dreams were vivid, but there was no enactment of dreams.

Mr. F. would get up at 6.45 am, but on occasions he stayed in bed until 1 pm. Other times, he was so tired that he needed to take a morning nap lasting several hours. There were no dreams associated with naps. His Epworth Sleepiness Scale score was 11 suggesting mild daytime sleepiness (see Appendix).

His past medical history was relevant for familial Charcot–Marie–Tooth disease (CMT). Medications included analgesics, an antidepressant and a statin. He had quit smoking marijuana and tobacco 4 months before.

On a review of systems, he complained of weakness of hands and legs. He had no difficulty swallowing.

Examination

The examination revealed a height of 1.73 m, a weight of 108 kg and a BMI of 36 kg/m^2. His hand grip was decreased bilaterally and dorsiflexion power was reduced in both feet. There was wasting of intrinsic muscles in both hands and in the anterior compartment of both legs. Sensory testing revealed decreased pin-prick perception in stocking and glove distribution and absent vibratory

Case Studies in Sleep Neurology: Common and Uncommon Presentations, ed. A. Culebras. Published by Cambridge University Press. © Cambridge University Press 2010.

perception in both legs. Deep tendon reflexes were absent. His gait was abnormal with moderate feet slapping; high arches were noted in both feet. Examination of the oropharynx revealed a Mallampati class 3 space. His pulse was regular and blood pressure was 140/90 mmHg. His neck circumference was 46.5 cm and waist circumference was 126 cm.

Special studies

Polysomnography (PSG) was carried out.

Question

Why does Mr. F. have severe sleep apnea?

Results of studies

The PSG evaluation showed abnormal results with an apnea–hypopnea index (AHI) of 77 events per hour of sleep (Figure 40.1). Most of the events were obstructive apneas and hypopneas. There were 532 arousals, of which 479 occurred with respiratory events, and 18 awakenings. Hemoglobin O_2 saturation levels showed a nadir of 75% in REM sleep, with 41.1% of the time showing O_2 saturation levels less than 90%. Snoring was of moderate loudness. In addition, there were 65 periodic leg movements of sleep (PLMS), many associated with respiratory events, with an index of 10 per hour of sleep. Thirty-four PLMS provoked arousals. Bruxism was audible, but difficult to distinguish from respiratory events. Sleep stages were normally proportioned relative to total sleep time; the EEG and the ECG were unremarkable. Sleeping supine did not affect the AHI.

Follow-up

A follow-up positive airway protocol (PAP) study showed a favorable response to the application of bilevel PAP with an inspiratory best pressure setting of 18 cmH$_2$O and an expiratory pressure of 14 cmH$_2$O (Figure 40.2). In addition, O_2 (2 l/min) was bled into the mask to maintain O_2 saturation levels above 88%. Tolerance was very good. His PLMS and restlessness decreased significantly, but bruxism continued to be audible. A significant REM-sleep rebound was noted (10% vs. 35% of total sleep time) with the application of bilevel PAP.

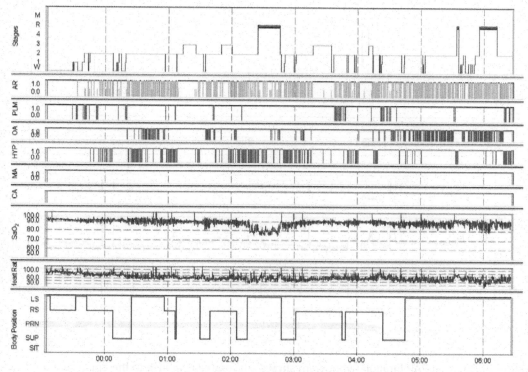

Figure 40.1 Hypnogram showing sleep apnea and hypopnea events with aggravation in REM sleep suggestive of associated mild diaphragmatic weakness. Stages: W, wake; R, REM; M, movement. AR, arousals; PLM, periodic leg movements; OA, obstructive apneas; HYP, hypopneas; MA, mixed apneas; CA, central apneas; SaO_2, hemoglobin saturation of O_2. Body position: LS, left side; RS, right side; PRN, prone; SUP, supine.

Diagnosis

The diagnosis was obstructive sleep apnea (OSA) of severe intensity (ICD9 Code 327.23) and Charcot–Marie–Tooth disease. In his case, risk factors for development of sleep apnea were age, obesity, a recent history of smoking and CMT. Patients with CMT frequently have sleep apnea as a result of widespread polyneuropathy affecting the function of oropharyngeal muscles and the diaphragm. ICSD-2 (AASM, 2005) classifies sleep-related hypoventilation/hypoxemia due to neuromuscular and chest-wall disorders under the heading "Sleep-related hypoventilation/hypoxemia due to medical conditions" within the larger category of "Sleep-related breathing disorders."

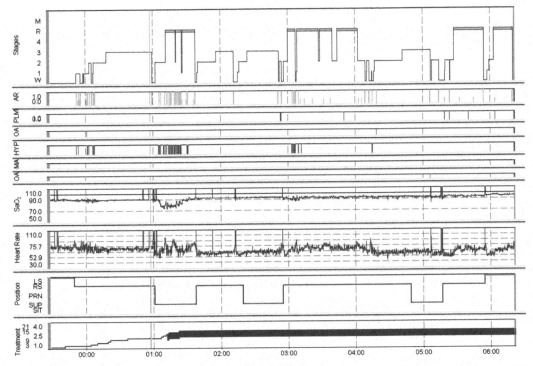

Figure 40.2 Bilevel PAP titration hypnogram shows a favorable response to the application of bilevel PAP at 18 cm of inspiratory and 14 cm of expiratory water pressure. Following the best pressure settings, the REM-sleep-related oximetry dip disappeared. Stages: W, wake; R, REM; M, movement. AR, arousals; PLM, periodic leg movements; OA, obstructive apneas; HYP, hypopneas; MA, mixed apneas; CA, central apneas; SaO_2, hemoglobin saturation of O_2. Body position: LS, left side; RS, right side; PRN, prone; SUP, supine. Treatment, initial CPAP followed by bilevel titration.

General remarks

Sleep-disordered breathing in neuromuscular disorders is secondary to involvement of the respiratory muscles, the neuromuscular junction, the phrenic and intercostal nerves or the lower motor neurons of the respiratory and oropharyngeal muscles. As a result of an abnormal ventilatory pump, patients are unable to maintain an arterial CO_2 pressure ($PaCO_2$) at or below 45 mmHg or normoxemia, particularly when asleep. The most common complaint is excessive daytime sleepiness (EDS) resulting from repeated arousals and sleep fragmentation caused by sleep-disordered breathing, hypoventilation, nocturnal hypoxemia or a combination of all three.

Patients with CMT have a high prevalence of obstructive sleep apnea syndrome (OSAS). One study showed that the severity of neuropathy and sleep apnea syndrome are highly correlated, and the authors suggested that pharyngeal neuropathy caused OSAS in these patients.

Phrenic nerve paralysis has also been reported in patients with CMT complicated with diabetes mellitus. Phrenic nerve damage leading to diaphragmatic paralysis may appear in polyneuropathies and in motor neuron disease. Unilateral phrenic nerve paralysis is asymptomatic, but bilateral paralysis is invariably symptomatic and may be life threatening. Bilateral paralysis leads to orthopnea with severe respiratory difficulty particularly in REM sleep when the only functional ventilatory muscle is the diaphragm. Undiagnosed bilateral diaphragmatic paralysis of any cause leads to acute cardiopulmonary failure and death.

Charcot–Marie–Tooth disease encompasses several inherited peripheral motor-sensory neuropathies and is one of the most common inherited neuromuscular diseases. The condition can be associated with restrictive pulmonary impairment, sleep apnea and vocal cord dysfunction. Restrictive pulmonary impairment has been described in association with phrenic nerve dysfunction, diaphragm muscle weakness or thoracic cage abnormalities. Vocal cord dysfunction, possibly due to laryngeal nerve involvement, is found in association with several CMT types and can often mimic asthma. Bilevel PAP may be more appropriate than continuous positive airway pressure (CPAP) for the treatment of sleep apnea in the individual with concomitant restrictive pulmonary impairment. The risk of progression to bilateral vocal cord dysfunction in CMT and the risk of aspiration with laryngeal neuropathy may limit the therapeutic options available for patients with vocal cord paralysis.

Pearls and gold

Sleep-disordered breathing in neuromuscular disorders is secondary to involvement of the respiratory muscles, the neuromuscular junction, the phrenic and intercostal nerves or the lower motor neurons of the respiratory and oropharyngeal muscles.

Patients with CMT have a high prevalence of OSAS.

Pharyngeal neuropathy may cause OSAS in patients with CMT.

Bilevel PAP may be more appropriate than CPAP for the treatment of sleep apnea in patients with concomitant restrictive pulmonary impairment due to weak muscles.

SUGGESTED READING

REVIEW

Culebras A. Sleep-disordered breathing in neuromuscular disease. *Sleep Med Clin* 2008; 3: 377–86.

GENERAL

Aboussouan LS, Lewis RA, Shy ME. Disorders of pulmonary function, sleep, and the upper airway in Charcot–Marie–Tooth disease. *Lung* 2007; 185: 1–7.

AASM (American Academy of Sleep Medicine). *International Classification of Sleep Disorders*, 2nd edn.: *Diagnostic and Coding Manual*. Westchester, Illinois: American Academy of Sleep Medicine, 2005.

Culebras A. REM-sleep related diaphragmatic insufficiency. *Neurology* 1998; **50**(Suppl. 4): 393–4.

Dematteis M, Pepin JL, Jeanmart M, *et al.* Charcot–Marie–Tooth disease and sleep apnoea syndrome: a family study. *Lancet* 2001; **357**: 267–72.

Appendix: Epworth Sleepiness Scale

0 = Would never doze
1 = Slight chance of dozing
2 = Moderate chance of dozing
3 = High chance of dozing

The Epworth Sleepiness Scale (ESS)

Sitting and reading	O_0	O_1	O_2	O_3
Watching television	O_0	O_1	O_2	O_3
Sitting inactive in a public place – for example, a theater or meeting	O_0	O_1	O_2	O_3
Lying down to rest in the afternoon when circumstances permit	O_0	O_1	O_2	O_3
Sitting and talking to someone	O_0	O_1	O_2	O_3
Sitting quietly after a lunch without alcohol	O_0	O_1	O_2	O_3
In a car, while stopped for a few minutes in traffic	O_0	O_1	O_2	O_3
As a passenger in a car for an hour without a break	O_0	O_1	O_2	O_3
CALCULATE	□			

1–10 Normal
10–15 Mild
15–20 Moderate
20–24 Severe

Index

Printed by Printforce, United Kingdom